This Gift of Health Provided by:

Advance Praise for
Love Is the Best Medicine™
for Dental Patients and the Dental Team

"For those in the field of dentistry, we're certain *Love Is the Best Medicine*™ *for Dental Patients and the Dental Team* will wow your soul and make it glow as you feel new pride in your profession. For those hundreds of millions of dental patients out there, we have no doubt you will thoroughly enjoy reading these true-life stories by—and about—the professionals who serve you in the dental office."

—**Mark Victor Hansen**
Co-creator, #1 *New York Times* Bestselling
Chicken Soup for the Soul® Series

"In one delightful book, the authors put the spotlight on what really counts in our work...and what really works in our lives. They make me proud to be part of the dental profession."

—**Steven L. Rasner, DMD, MAGD**

"This collection of short stories is like a tonic. After reading them, I am convinced that dentistry is unique among all of the health professions...."

—**J. Walter Coffey, DDS, FAGD, FASDC**
Editor
Newsletter for the Oklahoma Academy of General Dentistry

"It's easy to forget the human aspect of our profession. *Love Is the Best Medicine*™ *for Dental Patients and the Dental Team* reminds us of how we touch the lives of so many."

—**Danelle Fulawka, RDA**
2001 President
Canadian Dental Assistants' Association

"As a cosmetic dentist, I see people's lives transformed by dentistry every single day. Now there's an entire book, *Love Is the Best Medicine*™, dedicated to telling the world about the wonders of this magnificent profession, the joy it brings to patients, and the fulfillment it gives to every member of the dental team. I loved these stories!"

—**Thomas F. Trinkner, DDS**
Editor
The Journal of Cosmetic Dentistry
The official journal of the American Academy of Cosmetic Dentistry®

"*Love Is the Best Medicine*™ will warm the heart, tickle the funny-bone, and remind everyone why they love dentistry and the patients who make it fun and rewarding—an outstanding job by two fabulous writers who capture the essence of each story as if they were part of it. Don Dible and Rich Madow can rest assured that this book will surpass all others in its league. It's a perfect book for patients who refer, specialists looking for the perfect gift for the staff and dentists who refer to them, and the public in general."

—**Linda Miles**
CEO
Linda Miles and Associates

"There is no greater group of people than dental professionals. *Love Is the Best Medicine*™ is one more example of the love, care, and compassion that are evident parts of this amazing profession. The courage, strength, and faith exemplified throughout this book of human-interest stories is inspiring and validating. Thanks to all of you who shared your stories with us. Our lives are enriched as a result."

—**Cathy Jameson, PhD**
President
Jameson Management, Inc.

"Who knew? Who would have thought there could be a lovely, touching, humorous collection of stories about dentistry? Not me...until I served as a Story Contest Judge along with 84 other volunteers and helped with the selection of 100 stories from a field of 212 semi-finalists. The new book is titled *Love Is the Best Medicine*™ *for Dental Patients and the Dental Team.* Get your hands on a copy; you'll love it!"

—Sheridan Albert, DDS
Editor
The New York State Dental Journal

"The stories shared in *Love Is the Best Medicine*™ demonstrate dentists' talent, charm, and warmth. Too often dentists are depicted as insensitive or cold. Reading this book will shed new light on their capacity for compassion and love—truly the best medicine."

—Lauren Wood
Managing Editor
Mouth
The official journal of the American Student Dental Association

"Each day we are presented with opportunities to enhance lives through our work. These stories of hope and inspiration should motivate us all to build a legacy of caring for others."

—Linda Steel, DDS
National Chairperson
Give Back A Smile™ Foundation of the
American Academy of Cosmetic Dentistry®

"If you liked *Chicken Soup for the Dental Soul,* you'll LOVE *Love Is the Best Medicine*™ *for Dental Patients and the Dental Team.*"

—Jack Canfield
Co-creator of the 75 million copy
Chicken Soup for the Soul® series.

"A brand new smile can be life-changing. I was deeply touched by the impact dentistry has had on the lives of those whose stories appear in *Love Is the Best Medicine*™."

—William G. Dickerson, DDS, FAACD
Founder
The Las Vegas Institute for Advanced Dental Studies

"On days when it would be easy to just work on teeth, *Love Is the Best Medicine*™ is a great reminder that there's a real person attached! Dentistry...with a heart. That's what it's all about!"

—Walter Hailey
Founder
Dental Boot Kamp

"*Love Is the Best Medicine*™ is a breath of fresh air for dentists, their teams, and their patients...a delightful book, fun to read, and most uplifting."

—Peter E. Dawson, DDS
Founder and Director
Dawson Center for Advanced Dental Study

We would like to thank the following publishers and authors for permission to reprint the material indicated.

"Grandpa Browntooth." Reprinted by permission of Jeffrey C. Gray, DDS. © 2001 by Jeffrey C. Gray
"A Smile for Shelly." Reprinted by permission of Tom Orent, DMD. © 2001 by Tom Orent

(Continued on page 305)

LOVE IS THE BEST MEDICINE™
for Dental Patients and the Dental Team
published by DMD HOUSE

International Standard Book Number: 0-9713148-0-2
Library of Congress Control Number: 2001118470

Cover design, DMD HOUSE logo, and LOVE IS THE BEST MEDICINE™ series title logo created by Cha Designs, Redwood City, California 650.365.9446.

Heart and Rx logo designed by American Business Card, Scottsdale, Arizona 800.555.2234.

Front cover photography credits, top to bottom, left to right:
Father and son both brushing teeth, EyeWire Photography by arrangement with EyeWire, Inc.
Reflection of two girls brushing teeth, standing at bathroom sink, EyeWire Collection by arrangement with EyeWire, Inc. and Getty Images, Inc.
Lien Tran, Margaret McLoughlin, Katie Hurley, and Grant Palmer brushing teeth, photos by Allyson K. Hurley, DDS
Joseph and Rudy Diaz brushing teeth, photo by Cha Diaz
Dentist explaining how to brush teeth, photo by Scott T. Baxter by arrangement with PhotoDisk, Inc. and Getty Images, Inc.

For information, contact:
DMD HOUSE
29925 Rose Blossom Drive, Suite 300
Murrieta, CA 92563-4735

Contents

Acknowledgments   *Donald M. Dible* ....*xiii*
Introduction   *Richard H. Madow, DDS* ....*xviii*
Foreword   *Mark Victor Hansen* ....*xx*
Story Contests ....*xxiii*

1. HEARTWARMING SMILES
Grandpa Browntooth *Jeffrey C. Gray, DDS* 2
A Smile for Shelly   *Tom Orent, DMD* 6
New Smile, New Life!   *Rhonda R. Savage, DDS* 9
The Biggest Smile   *Cheryl Lee Willett, DDS, MS* 12
Jane and the Tetracycline Stain
          Jeffrey M. Galler, DDS, MAGD 14
Paid in Full *J. Walter Coffey, DDS, FAGD, FASDC* 16

2. RAISING SELF-ESTEEM
Pat's Final Gift   *Richard H. Madow, DDS* 20
Gerhardt and Edith   *Sue O'Brien, RDH* 25
Never Too Late   *A.T. Williams, DDS* 27
The Hidden Smile   *Jackie Lais, CDA, CDPMA* 29
A Good Boy   *Robert C. Smithwick, DDS, FACD* 32
Sammy   *D. Michael Hart, DDS, FAGD, MAGD* 35
Sheila's Diastema   *Jeffrey M. Galler, DDS, MAGD*............39
Teeth Maketh the Man   *Kenneth Grubbs, DDS* 41
Temp Rewards   *Karen L. Hart-Sabol, RDH* 43
I Feel Rich!   *Donald L. Gary, DDS, FAGD* 47
Credit Report   *Amy M. McLamb* 49

3. COMPASSION AND KINDNESS
The Farnham Legacy   *Bert F. Engstrom, DMD* 54
Full Circle   *Lisa M. Wendell, DMD* 56
One Winter   *Steven Novick, DDS* 59
Steak for the Colonel   *Christopher Freyermuth, DMD*.........63

Alice *Marla Leibfried, CDA* 67
On Call for Christmas *Thomas G. Dwyer, DDS, MS* 69
Home for Christmas Dinner
    Pamela Arbuckle Alston, DDS, FACD 72
Sarah *Sharon Louise Melanson, RDH* 75
Children of Bosnia *Eric B. Wall, DDS* 77
Steve *Debby Kurtz-Weidinger, RDH, MEd* 80
Seek and Ye Shall Find *Richard L. Parker, DDS, MS* 84

4. A FULFILLING CAREER
Sweet Sixteen *Rudi Neumarker, DDS* 88
Giving and Receiving *Becky Sroda, RDH, MS* 92
You *Do* Make a Difference! *Danelle Fulawka, RDA* 95
A Mother's Faith *Janice M. Dionis, RDH* 97
The Baby Business *Sheila Hall, DDS* 101
A Dedicated Dental Assistant *Bess Reeverts CDA, RDA* ..104
Friendship *Sandra C. Nelson, RDH, BS, LAP* 106
Northwest Flight 255 *Robert E. Lavine, DDS* 108

5. MISSION: POSSIBLE
The Power of Faith *Paul A. Bonstead, DDS* 114
Kisses from Madagascar *Elizabeth A. Brandenburg, DA* ..118
Saving a Life *Sherwin R. Shinn, DDS* 121
Dental Images *Cathy Milejczak, CDA, RDH, BHS* 124
National Geographic *Julie Burton, RDH* 126
Little Shoes *Mary M. O'Connor, DDS* 129
Flying Doctors *Adrian D. Fenderson, DDS* 131

6. GOLDEN YEARS
Keepsake Crown *John McCormack, DDS* 138
The Colonel *Sue O'Brien, RDH* 141
Fish Story *Leanne Haynes, RDH, BS* 144
Questionnaire *Gregory R. Johnson, DDS* 146
Curing Cancer *Clyde T. Padgett, Jr., DDS* 147
Full-Service Station *Nancy Roe-Pimm, RDH* 150
Sweet Surrender *Robin Brenner, RDH* 153

Sharing   *Robert F. Weed, DDS*...155
My Valentine   *Mary S. Pelletier, RDH, BS*...........................157
Song of Love   *Mary Jo Pletz, RDH* 160

7. LITTLE SURPRISES

Expensive Diet   *Stanley J. Larsen, DDS* 164
Wasted Effort   *Ira Marder, DDS, FAGD* 165
Family Dentistry   *Harry T. Keyes, DDS*.............................166
Soft Diet   *Robert E. Riddle, DDS*...................................167
Marital Status   *Mohamed Hussein, DDS*...........................168
Shhhhhhhhhh!   *Robert Reyto, DDS, FAACD* 169
Bloodcurdling Screams
        Jeffrey M. Galler, DDS, MAGD 171
Easy Choice   *Linda L. Miles, CSP, CMC*...........................174
Cutting Confusion   *David Zamboni, RDH, BS* 176
Shattered Confidence   *Linda Williams, RDH* 178
Survival Instinct   *Mitchell J. Burgin, DDS*..........................179
My Young Dental Assistant   *Judee Limardi, RDH*..............180
Fashion Statement   *Ann Madigan, DMD, MSc*..................182

8. TOOTH FAIRY STORIES

The Tooth Fairy   *Nancy Roe-Pimm, RDH* 186
Notes from the Tooth Fairy   *Shari Caplan, RDH* 188
Mom, Are You Listening?
        Cathy Milejczak, CDA, RDH, BHS 190
Expensive Precedent   *Cheryl Lee Willett, DDS, MS* 191
A Grain of Tooth   *Diane Brucato-Thomas, RDH, EF, BS*....192

9. LEARNING FROM OUR PATIENTS

Sam Eagle   *Helen Jasnosz, DDS* 196
Life Lessons   *Kathleen E. Banas, RDH* 200
Little Billy   *Sherwin R. Shinn, DDS*...................................204
Punctured Ego   *Robert E. Lavine, DDS*.............................209
Dental Détente   *Richard L. Plasch, DDS, FAGD*................211
A Bad Day   *Mary Cole, RDH*...213
He Cared   *John R. Grasso, DDS* 215

10. THANK YOU, *THANK YOU!*

Oh, I Have a Terrible Pain in My Head!
    Naomi Rhode, RDH, CSP, CPAE..............................218
No Charge, Professor
    Andrew Christopher, BS, DDS, MHA, FICD 222
Agnes and Her Precious Gift   *Robert J. Harland, DMD* 224
The Art of Appreciation   *Ian W. Tester, DDS*......................226
Once Again, Thank You   *Daniel E. White, DDS*.................228
A Thousand Hugs   *Jackie S. Perry, RDH, BSDH*.................230
A Letter for My Father   *S.G. Cooley* 232

11. BEYOND DENTISTRY

We Care   *Joanne Iannone Sheehan, RDH* 236
Oklahoma Healing   *April Klepper, RDH* 239
Nicky   *Mandy Hayre-Dhasi, RDH, BDSc, PID* 242
Cradling People in My Lap   *Noel Brandon-Kelsch, RDH* ..246
Blessed Event   *Sherrie L. Frame, RDH* 249
Puppy Therapy   *Deborah D. Landis, RDH* 252
Eighteen Months   *Jane Weiner, RDH* 254
Golfer's Last Wish   *Allyson K. Hurley, DDS, MAGD, AACD* ..256

12. OUTSIDE THE BOX

Today Is a Gift   *Cathy Jameson, PhD* 260
Taking a Bite Out of Crime   *Christy King, RDH* 265
Bomb Squad   *Charles S. Horn, III, DDS*.............................268
Sammy, Poor Sammy   *Jeffrey M. Galler, DDS, MAGD* 270
Eye Teeth   *Betty Moss, CDA* 273
Blurred Vision   *Ethel Wolff, RDH* 274
Live the Dream   *Steven L. Rasner, DMD, MAGD* 276

Story Contest for the Sequel to This Book 279
Giving Back to the Community 281
Meet the Co-authors...284
Meet the Contributors 286

Acknowledgments

If you think about the last blockbuster movie you saw, you'll remember that the credits seemed to roll on forever. In preparing for the huge task of acknowledging everyone who helped create this book, we've discovered that the number is more than 500! In fairness to our readers, it's simply not appropriate to cite every single person. Instead, the list will be limited to those who had major roles in bringing *Love Is the Best Medicine*™ *for Dental Patients and the Dental Team* to print.

Without the support of my wife, Alice, this book would not exist. At various times she functioned as a proofreader, critic, design consultant, cheerleader, and master of many mundane-but-important tasks too numerous to mention. Additionally, in the last month of production the Dibles relocated their home office some 450 miles to the south, from the San Francisco Bay Area to the city of Murrieta, California, located in the Temecula Valley north of San Diego. Alice was totally responsible for orchestrating the move and working with the builder of our new home to make it ready for occupancy, thus ensuring no slippage in the tight production schedule for this book. Thank you, Sweetheart. I love you.

To my co-author, Dr. Richard H. Madow, whose phenomenal knowledge of the dental profession and the people in it has proven invaluable in securing wonderful stories from a number of leaders in the field. My daily email correspondence with him has provided a wealth of guidance, humor, and inspiration. Responsible for editing *The Richards Report*—an enormously popular newsletter serving the dental community, and putting together the annual Richards Report Super Fall Seminar—truly The Best Seminar Ever (T.B.S.E.)—he always managed to find time to work on this project when I needed his help. Thank you for your major contributions, Rich!

To S.G. Cooley, a gifted writer and developmental editor in Washington State. Scherry assists emerging authors in bringing out the best in their stories and shepherded the work of a dozen whose material appears in this book. The joint effort that made this possible was a series of three-part collaborations between publisher, editor, and writer. A good editor's work is seamless; it disappears between the lines. Scherry, for the quality of your work—warmly acknowledged by each of the authors with whom you collaborated—many thanks!

To Mark Victor Hansen and Jack Canfield, co-creators of the Chicken Soup for the Soul® series, for their invitation to me to co-author *Chicken Soup for the Dental Soul*. My experience on that book proved invaluable in producing *Love Is the Best Medicine™ for Dental Patients and the Dental Team*.

To my dentist of almost 30 years, Dr. Rudi Neumarker, with whom I had several lunches at a restaurant on the Stanford University campus across the street from his office. It was during these meals that he shared his recommendations and insights into the dental profession. These get-togethers also provided the opportunity for me to interview the good doctor and elicit his personal story, "Sweet Sixteen," appearing here.

To Linda L. Miles, CSP, CMC, CEO of Linda Miles and Associates and author of "Easy Choice," who referred more than 20 manuscripts to us. Our Story Contest Judges selected many of those stories for publication in *Love Is the Best Medicine™ for Dental Patients and the Dental Team*.

This list of acknowledgments would not be complete without recognizing the vitally important support of the many newsletters, bulletins, magazines, and journals serving the dental profession whose editors were kind enough to bring our Story Contest to the attention of their members and subscribers. I would especially like to thank Dr. Joe Blaes, editor of *Dental Economics*, and Mark Hartley, editor of *RDH* magazine, for their ongoing support of the book publishing and distribution activities of DMD House.

To the winners of our Story Contest: Jeffrey C. Gray, DDS, author of "Grandpa Browntooth," grand prize recipient for the best story written by a dentist; Joanne Iannone Sheehan, RDH, author of "We Care," and Diane Brucato-Thomas, RDH, EF, BS, author of "A Grain of Tooth," who will share the grand prize for best story written by a dental hygienist; Elizabeth A. Brandenburg, DA, author of "Kisses from Madagascar," grand prize winner for best story written by a dental assistant; and Jackie Lais, CDA, CDPMA, author of "The Hidden Smile," and Amy McLamb, author of "Credit Report," who will share the grand prize for best story written by a dental practice administrator.

To Rochelle Pennington, co-author of *Highlighted in Yellow*—with H. Jackson Brown, Jr., author of the bestselling *Life's Little Instruction Book*® series. Rochelle has an extraordinary interest in quotations and supplied most of those printed in *Love Is the Best Medicine*™ *for Dental Patients and the Dental Team*. Her work has added spice and richness to our story mix. Thank you, Shelly.

To Cha Diaz who not only designed the impressive jacket of this book but also supplied the front cover photograph of her toothbrushing sons, Joseph and Rudy. And to Dr. Allyson K. Hurley, author of "Golfer's Last Wish" published here, who was kind enough to supply photographs of four of her patients brushing their teeth. Those pictures—including one of her daughter, Katie Hurley—grace our front cover.

To our 85 Story Contest Judges: Sheridan Albert, DDS; R. Scott Anderson, DMD; Mary Backstrom; Kay L. Bandle, RDH; Karen Bateman, RDH; Josette Beach, RDH, MS; Anne Bettiol, PDA; Paul Bonstead, DDS; Noel Brandon-Kelsch, RDH; Pat Bychowski; Mary Christofferson, CDA, EFDA; Paul H. Coleman, DMD; Annemarie Condito, CDA, RDA; Margaret L. Conrad, RDH, BS; Janet Crain, DMD; Sandy Darling; Carolyn J. Davis, CDA; Sherry Delaney; Dorothy Dixon, RDH; Jodi D. Dotson, DMD; Sharon Efron, RDH; Jan Eygendaal, CDA, BS; Adrian D. Fenderson, DDS; Karen D. Foster; Sandi Gallagher, CDA; Susan Ballou Gibson, DMD, MSD; Cindy L. Godfrey, RDH; Mary Lou

Goforth; Oscar Goren, DMD; Sarah L. Gresko, CDA, RDA; Mary Gum, RDA; Anne Gwozdek, RDH; Karen L. Hart-Sabol, RDH; Sue Hauenstein, CDA; Cheryl Herrmann, RDH; Gary E. Heyamoto, DDS, FAGD; Barbara A. Hickey, COA; James L. Hillman, DMD; Fran Holbrook, CDA; Shelli Johnson, CDA; Marthenia Jones; Jackie Lais, CDA, CDPMA; Robert E. Lavine, DDS; Marjean Lehman; Marla Leibfried, CDA; Terry Lepine; Genna Leutzinger; Richard H. Madow, DDS; Sharyn Markus; Carol A. Martin, RDH; Denise Maus, RDH; Gregory V. McGowan, DDS; Denise McIntire, CDA; Cathy Meachum, RDH; David J. Mikulencak, DDS; Cathy Milejczak, CDA, RDH, BHS; Bill H. Molsberry, DDS; Pat Mueller, CDA, RDA; Judy Nist, RDH; Mary M. O'Connor, DDS; Mary S. Pelletier, RDH, BS; Maria Perno, RDH, MS; Connie Pero-Fox, CDA; Jackie S. Perry, RDH, BSDH; Wendy Pio, RDA; Richard L. Plasch, DDS, FAGD; Diane Proto, RDA; Steven C. Reynolds, DDS; Cynthia A. Rider, DMD; Susan Ryals, RDH; Denise Rysz, RDH, BHS; Paul Schlesinger; Sherry Smith; Kathleen A. Stambaugh, DDS; Teri Steinberg, DDS; Laura Szlanfucht, RDH; Julie Taucher, RDH; Sandy Tesch, RDH; Ian W. Tester, DDS; Andrew Toeman, DDS; Catherine L. Tonne; Lauren Waggoner; Carol A. Walsh, CDA, CDPMA; Carol Ann Walsh, CDA; Joan Weiner; and Nancy Zolan, RDH each of who somehow found the time in their busy schedules as dentists, dental hygienists, dental assistants, and patients to read—and grade—212 semifinalist manuscripts from which the stories in this book were selected.

To Chester J. Zhivanos whose command of the English language—especially in matters of grammar and punctuation—is precise and elegant. In the space of a week, Chester took hundreds of pages of our final manuscript and went over them with meticulous care to help us minimize embarrassing errors. I take full responsibility for any lapses in correcting problems he flagged with his busy, bright red pencil.

At the time our Story Contest was announced, we also requested that folks send us recommendations for dental-related cartoons. In response, we received material from Gabriele M.

Hamm, CDPMA; Christopher Kleber, DDS, MAGD (a phenomenal collection of more than 100 newspaper and magazine clippings); Michael A. Peele, DDS (an entire bookful) to whom I was referred by Donald L. Gary, DDS; Mitchell J. Burgin, DDS; Mary Christofferson, CDA, EFDA; Robbie L. Tanner, EFDA; Crystal Fields-Oxendine; Pamela Skehan; Ruth Ludeman; and Joseph Bore. The odd thing is that almost every cartoon submitted portrayed dentistry in a negative way. In the four years I've worked on the production of *Chicken Soup for the Dental Soul* and *Love Is the Best Medicine™ for Dental Patients and the Dental Team,* I have come to appreciate that dentistry is a warm and caring profession and that those who work in it are deeply committed to patient wellbeing. Sadly, today's cartoonists don't seem to understand this. As our press deadline drew near and the tiny inventory of usable cartoons was assessed, the decision was made not to use *any* rather than delay publication with an ongoing search for material that accurately characterizes this wonderful profession.

To Andrew Simms of Datantics whose knowledgeable consulting—onsite and by phone—kept the many devices in my two-computer network humming harmoniously.

To my sister, Calder Lowe, and to Shah Carlo Varahramyan, Executive Vice President of American Business Card, for their sustained encouragement over the years.

To those whom I have failed to acknowledge, either because of the limitations of space or my inability to keep track of everyone, I apologize. No slight was intended. You know who you are and can take great pride in your role in the creation of *Love Is the Best Medicine™ for Dental Patients and the Dental Team.*

—Don Dible
Murrieta, California
2001

Introduction

In 1980, upon entering the freshman class at the University of Maryland School of Dentistry, I was, as the saying goes, totally clueless. As with most first-year dental students, I had good grades in college in a difficult major (microbiology in my case), an ability to interview well, probably some luck, and absolutely no idea whatsoever what it would be like to provide healthcare to a fellow human being, run a business, manage a staff, and be, as all dentists are, Michelangelo on the head of a pin—a pin that is moving, sometimes uncomfortable, and always wanting to exit as quickly as possible.

Dentistry can be a tough, sometimes grueling, profession. Even the best patients would rather be somewhere else—and don't hesitate to tell you so. But that is the main reason why this book is so special. The stories were contributed by some of the greatest people in the world—dental assistants, dental hygienists, dental office staff, dentists themselves, and dental patients. All of these exceptional people know that between scheduling nightmares, fighting insurance companies, trying to provide excellent treatment when conditions are less than ideal, and putting up with patients who don't floss (that's 98% of us!), there is no greater feeling than allowing someone to eat better and be more comfortable, and the most fun thing of all—providing someone with a great big beautiful smile.

The stories contained in this book tell of some amazing accomplishments and some extraordinary people—some of whose names we've changed to protect their privacy. But the stories also tell of many minor miracles—the touching of a child's heart, a little chuckle during a hard day, a ray of hope where none previously existed, a chance to give a well-deserved thank-you. Some stories will bring a laugh, and more than a few will bring tears. But each and every story will bring a smile. And that's what we dentists are all about. So pull up a chair, a hammock, or my favorite, a floor—and get ready to enjoy the many reasons why it is so true that *Love Is the Best Medicine*™.

It wouldn't be fair of me to end this Introduction without thanking a few special people. Don Dible—you have done an incredible job of putting this project together. You are an inspiration! Thanks to my parents, Lois and Selvin Madow, for raising me and for always being there. Thanks to my brother Marshall for being a great brother and friend, for being so much fun to work with, and for always coming up with the best trivia questions. Thanks to my brother Dave, also a great brother and friend, for the incredible, unpredictable, and sometimes outrageous journey we have taken together since founding The Madow Group over a decade ago. Thanks to my wife, Anne, and my children, Michelle and Steven, for being the best, most supportive, loving, and most fun family anybody could ever want. You guys are as great as side two of *Abbey Road*. And thanks to all of my other family and friends, whose mention would put me over the word limit that Chief Dible has imposed!

Enjoy this book, and may your smiles be contagious.

—Richard Madow
Owings Mills, Maryland
2001

Foreword

I've enjoyed reading Don Dible's motivational and self-help books for more than 25 years. In his work, you will discover an inspiring writer and a superb storyteller. As an editor, Don never fails to bring out the best in any story. In his latest book, *Love Is the Best Medicine*™ *for Dental Patients and the Dental Team*, Don has collaborated with hundreds of dental professionals in bringing you inspiring and heartwarming behind-the-scenes insights into the practice of dentistry.

As co-creators of the *Chicken Soup for the Soul*® series, my longtime friend, Jack Canfield, and I were honored to have Don help us put together *Chicken Soup for the Dental Soul*. With more than 100,000 copies in print, that book is a roaring success with dentists, dental hygienists, dental assistants, members of the dental office staff, and an increasing number of dental patients. *Dental Soul* is unquestionably the bestselling nonfiction, nontechnical dental book of all time. I feel strongly—and have no doubt—that *Love Is the Best Medicine*™ will ultimately share in that publishing success.

Jack Canfield and I sincerely believe that stories are—and always have been—the best enrollment tool on the planet. The stories in *Chicken Soup for the Dental Soul* and *Love Is the Best Medicine*™ *for Dental Patients and the Dental Team* sneak up on you. They get inside you. And they make you receptive to the message: "I *can* eradicate my fear of going to the dentist," "I *can* feel comfortable during the dental procedure," and "I *can* leave the dental office with greatly improved oral health." Furthermore, it is a proven fact that good oral hygiene vastly improves the quality of life and enhances longevity.

Through *Dental Soul* and *Love Is the Best Medicine*™, Don has shown that dental professionals are caring, loving, and sometimes even cuddly people. Unfortunately, the media have portrayed most dentists as purveyors of anguish, pain, and torment. (Remember *Marathon Man* or *The Little Shop of Horrors?*) The reality is that dentists minimize pain and maximize oral health. Solid clinical evidence shows conclusively that ignoring your teeth and avoiding the dentist are guaranteed to result in dental problems—along with the discomfort and ill health associated with them.

For those in the field of dentistry, we're certain *Love Is the Best Medicine*™ *for Dental Patients and the Dental Team* will wow your soul and make it glow as you feel new pride in your profession. For those hundreds of millions of dental patients out there, we have no doubt you will thoroughly enjoy reading these true-life stories by—and about—the professionals who serve you in the dental office.

As a great fan of dentistry—and especially my own dentist, Dr. Mark Daniels of Huntington Beach, California—I know that *Love Is the Best Medicine*™ *for Dental Patients and the Dental Team* is going to help eradicate dental phobia, anesthetize oral pain, and ultimately improve the general health of tens of thousands—maybe even millions—of dental patients. It will put big, happy smiles on the faces of dental professionals and dental patients alike, each of whom will thank Don and his co-authors in their prayers.

Happy Thinking.

—Mark Victor Hansen, Co-creator
#1 *New York Times* Bestselling
Chicken Soup for the Soul® Series

Story Contests

Do you have a great story you'd like to have published in a future volume of the LOVE IS THE BEST MEDICINE™ series? We are looking for true stories similar in appeal to those in this book and are conducting a series of story contests.

For each title, one or more grand prizes of $1,000 will be awarded to selected authors whose stories are published. *Only a very small percentage of those authors whose stories are selected will receive a grand prize.* (A total of four grand prizes were shared among six prizewinners in this book.) Other authors whose stories are accepted each receive compensation in the form of 20 copies of the book. For this compensation, authors agree to provide DMD House with the non-exclusive rights to publish their stories. For a full set of contest rules and submission deadlines for various titles, see our website.

After reading this book, you should have a good idea of the type of material we'd like to receive. Forthcoming books will include editions on Southern Gospel Music, weddings, and of course, *Love Is the Best Medicine™ for Dental Patients and the Dental Team—Volume Two.* Send non-returnable submissions to:

Story Contest Editor
DMD House
29925 Rose Blossom Drive, Suite 300
Murrieta, CA 92563-4735 USA
Email: dondible@dmdhouse.net
Fax: 909.698.0180
Website: www.dmdhouse.net

All non-returnable submissions should include the name, address, phone number, and email address (if you have one) of the author. A postcard will be sent acknowledging receipt of all materials. Please keep a copy of all submissions for your files.

Love cures people—
both the ones who give it
and the ones who receive it.

—Karl A. Menninger, MD
Founder, The Menninger Clinic
University of Missouri

1

HEARTWARMING SMILES

*It is almost impossible
to smile on the outside
without feeling better
on the inside.*

—Anonymous

Grandpa Browntooth

Let every nation know, whether it wishes us well or ill,
that we shall pay any price, bear any burden,
meet any hardship, and oppose any foe
to assure the survival and the success of liberty.

—John F. Kennedy

 everal years ago a new patient, Russell, was referred to our practice. I was immediately struck by his incredibly happy demeanor and wonderful attitude. After a few visits, it came out that Russ was one of the unfortunate few who led the assault on the beaches of Normandy, "D-Day," in World War II. Wounded during the invasion, he was awarded a Purple Heart. A determined soldier, he went on to fight for six more months until he was gravely wounded in the Battle of the Bulge while single-handedly saving his entire company from a German ambush. It seems Russ charged up a hill under heavy fire, found an abandoned bazooka, and took out a deadly machine-gun nest that had pinned down his platoon. He won the Bronze Star that day and a second Purple Heart for his actions.

While chatting with Russ during a subsequent appointment, I asked him a question that I ask all my patients sooner or later: "If I had a magic wand, what could I do to make you happy?" While this question is motivated as much by curiosity as anything else, I try to be of help where and when I can.

"Oh, Dr. Gray, I could never afford it, but I would love for my front teeth not to be brown. My grandkids call me 'Grandpa Browntooth.' "

Since I'm the intensely patriotic type, I knew at that instant exactly what would happen. I told Russ that in honor of his service to our country, he would have matching front teeth—and that, in my book, he had already paid for the procedure on the Normandy coast all those years ago.

Never have I enjoyed dentistry, or life, as much as when I saw his face light up the moment he gazed at his new smile for the first time. What made that experience even more satisfying was when—later that day—his daughter, in tears, called to thank me. Since then, Russ and I have become great friends, and he is almost a second Dad to me.

Here is the truly amazing part of the story. Due to the usual government errors, it was nearly 50 years after D-Day before Russ received his medals! At the insistence of his daughter, he had written the necessary letters to Washington and finally received his due: three Purple Hearts, a Combat Infantry Badge, and, of course, the Bronze Star along with numerous other decorations. Since Russ received his medals around the time of the release of the movie "Saving Private Ryan," I asked if he would mind sharing more of his story for our practice newsletter. He agreed as long as I didn't make him out to be some kind of hero.

We talked and cried for nearly two hours, as he had not spoken of those war memories for nearly 50 years. Even his wife, who lovingly patted his hand from time to time during the interview, couldn't believe some of his recollections. His closing statement was that, although he was proud of his Bronze Star, the medals that meant the most were his Combat Infantry Badge and his first Purple Heart. These symbols commemorated the fact that he was part of the action on D-Day. Most of all, these medals honored his reverence for those who gave their lives for the freedom we now enjoy. I was truly moved by what Russ had said—and by what those Americans had done.

everal days later, I arrived at the office to find a simple package wrapped in green paper. Being in a hurry I wasn't sure I had time to look at the new arrival, but something drew me to it. When I saw the box was from Russ, my hands began to tremble. As I peeled back the paper, tears filled my eyes—just as they do now while I record those events. In that small box was a gift incredibly special—from a man who had already given me so much. Through my tears, I saw that the box contained his Combat Infantry Badge and a Purple Heart from WWII. To these items, Russ had added a small plaque that said, "To Dr. Gray, A Great Human Being, From An Old Soldier." I was stunned. For a few minutes, I had trouble breathing. To think that something as simple as spending a couple of hours bonding his front teeth and then listening to his story could move a man to such gratitude. He was delighted that his grandkids just called him Grandpa now.

Along with the medals and personalized plaque, Russ enclosed the following letter:

Dear Dr. Gray,

At a point in our history when so many people have no time for today and think only of tomorrow, it is refreshing to find someone who has a sincere and genuine interest in those who sacrificed so much to ensure the freedom that we enjoy. I would like you to accept this gift on behalf of all my comrades, those who survived and those who never had a chance to enjoy the freedom for which they gave their lives.

Keep well, and may God be with you and yours always.

Sincerely,

Russell

On that note: God Bless Dentistry, and may He continue to bless the U.S.A.! ❤

—Jeffrey C. Gray, DDS

A Smile for Shelly

his is a true account of hope and recovery, and the tenderness of love between mother and child. About a young woman emerging from a dark cocoon, this isn't pretty. But it is lovely. Here is Deborah's story....

Our first meeting took place on a cold New England morning. Although most initial visits start with a patient's medical and dental histories, this case was different. Deborah, 32, just looked down at her feet and cried. She looked everywhere but at me, and rarely spoke.

She had been in an abusive relationship for more than ten years: physical violence and emotional torture. Her husband had convinced her that she was hideous, ugly...and that she would always be ugly. He had gained complete control of her mind.

And there was insidious, long-term neglect. Over the years her husband would visit the dentist. But there was never any money spent on Deborah's dental care. When she had dental emergencies, her husband filled cavities and extracted her teeth, right there in the house. After a decade of virtual imprisonment in her own home, Deborah escaped.

That's when I met her. As a cosmetic dentist, I partner with the Give Back A Smile™ program, providing dental services to victims of domestic violence. GBAS is the fulfilled dream of Dr. Wynn Okuda, a leader in the American Academy of Cosmetic Dentistry. Participating dentists restore teeth damaged by physical abuse, rebuilding a patient's confidence and self-respect.

The GBAS orientation is clinically thorough. But nothing prepared me for the seriousness of Deborah's condition. Nothing.

All of her top front teeth were decayed down to the gumline. Her back teeth were in a similar state. The fractures and deterioration she lived with were an obvious source of chronic pain.

But there was a bright side. She was out of the abusive situation—one of the GBAS prerequisites for participation in the program. She was taking better care of herself in every respect. Deborah was beginning—for the first time in a very long time—to see herself in a positive light.

Old habits, though, are tough to break. She apologized for everything, even simple things beyond her control. If she was faced to the left, and I asked her to turn slightly toward me on the right, she would apologize for being in *the wrong position.* It was scary to think of the emotional nightmare that had conditioned such an unnatural response.

So I made a deal with Deborah. I would fix her teeth only if she promised to stop apologizing. The compulsion to apologize was so deeply ingrained that when she did it *anyway*, she would apologize *again* for messing up! That kind of broke the tension, as she eventually saw the humorous irony in apologizing for an apology.

Because of the severity of dental trauma and neglect, this case required many visits. While we worked on Deborah, there was another family member present, her three-year-old daughter. Shelly was cute as a button and good as gold. While I worked on her mother, she would play in the corner of the treatment room, and we hardly knew she was there. Once in a while, she'd climb into the chair and snuggle down in mom's lap during the long treatments.

 will never forget the day we started to rebuild Deborah's smile. The decay was gone, and root canal treatments had been performed on most of her teeth. It was time to begin the process of restoration. During an afternoon-long appointment, I placed temporary crowns on every top front tooth.

When I was finished, I handed Deborah a mirror while everyone on my staff and I watched anxiously.

Everyone but little Shelly. Grinning from ear to ear, she climbed into her mother's lap. Her hands reached for Deborah's mouth, and she ran her tiny fingertips over the smooth, clean teeth.

I was delightfully puzzled by the reaction, and my face clearly telegraphed my lack of understanding to Deborah.

She looked up at me through fresh, happy tears, and broke the silence:

"Doctor, this is the first time Shelly's ever seen me smile!" ♥

—Tom Orent, DMD

If you know a survivor of domestic violence
in need of help from the
Give Back A Smile™ Program,
contact:

The American Academy of Cosmetic Dentistry®
1-800-543-9220
www.aacd.com

New Smile, New Life!

s a dental student, you will always remember your first restorative patient. You will also always remember your fourth-year esthetic patient. At my dental school, your fourth-year esthetic patient could be a patient who needed a fixed bridge, veneers, crowns, or any combination of treatments.

I met Kurt, my fourth-year esthetic patient, early in my last year of dental school. He was from Germany—a tall, dark-haired man with a long mustache. He had an extremely shy demeanor and wouldn't look at me when we met. Kurt walked with his head down, shoulders hunched, and a look of defeat in his eyes. It took a number of visits before he opened up to me.

Kurt told me he had been in our country only a few days when he was mugged in an alleyway in a big city. He lost three front teeth at the hands of his assailants when he was hit in the face with a steel bar. Many years had passed since he was mugged. It had taken him more than a decade of menial labor before he could save enough money to come to the dental school for treatment. I talked with him about his options, which included implants, fixed bridgework, and a removable prosthesis.

To me, a young dentist at the time, it seemed strangely clinical to talk with Kurt about options when the replacement of his teeth was a very personal matter. It was hard to talk to him about options and financial arrangements while he stared silently at the ground. He told me he had limited finances but wanted to replace the lost teeth with a permanent restoration—not something removable. He understood that a partial denture is an appliance that would need to be removed nightly with his fingers. To him, this wasn't an acceptable replacement for his missing teeth. So I made him a cemented fixed bridge that would never need to be removed.

Kurt and I spent many visits together as I tried to restore his teeth to a more natural appearance. Finally, the day had come to put his new bridgework in permanently. I gave him a mirror and held my breath, hoping he would be happy with the final work.

Kurt didn't say a word. He simply placed the mirror in his lap with the reflective side down and looked off into the distance. I couldn't tell if he liked the work or not. I was at a loss. I let him sit in silence for a bit, then asked if he liked the bridge. He gave me a solemn nod. Having secured my patient's approval, I bonded the bridgework with cement; and he left without saying a word. I felt empty.

everal weeks later, Kurt came back for his follow-up visit. I was worried when I went out to the large dental school reception area because I didn't see him. He had been punctual for all his other dental appointments, and I was concerned since the follow-up appointment was a big part of our fourth-year treatment. Finally, from the back of the room, a man stood up—it was Kurt. I hadn't recognized him! He had shaved off his mustache, wore a big grin, looked me directly in the eye, and walked with a straight back. Gone were the shy, defeated look and the hunched shoulders. I was ecstatic!

I had seen a transformation—created by my work. To this day, Kurt's transformation continues to motivate me as an esthetically conscious dentist; and for this I will be forever grateful to him. Kurt went on in life to become a successful businessman, keeping in touch with me by mail and telephone through the years. The creation of a beautiful smile had changed his life, his confidence, and his attitude. ❤

—Rhonda R. Savage, DDS

The Biggest Smile

ally was adopted by American parents when she was six months old. Her Eastern European biological family had given up the child because of her physical differences—she had Ectrodactyly Ectodermal Dysplasia with Clefting Syndrome. In simple terms, Sally had multiple deformities associated with her hair, eyes, nose, mouth, glands, hands, and feet. Weighing only 11 pounds when she arrived in the United States, the child faced multiple surgeries and hospitalizations.

I met Sally for the first time when she was six years of age. At that first meeting I observed a child the size of an average three-year-old. Her eyes looked at me from under half-closed, protective eyelids. As I returned her gaze, I noticed a head adorned with scattered wisps of hair, two hands and two feet that had lobster-claw-like deformities, a surgically repaired nose, and a mouth furnished with almost no teeth. She had great difficulty with speech due to her lack of teeth, multiple oral and nasal defects, and previous attempts at surgical repair. What Sally also had was the biggest smile you could imagine. Despite all of her differences, she was a very loving and extremely happy child.

Sally's parents informed me at that first visit that they would never suggest changing one thing about her unless she asked to have different teeth, or a wig, or different hands and feet. About six months after that initial meeting, I received a call from Sally's mother. She wanted to know if I could make her daughter "some teeth." She continued by telling me that while they were visiting a pumpkin patch, another little girl began screaming in Sally's face. The stranger yelled to her own mother, *"Mommy, look at this girl! She doesn't have eyes or teeth! Look at her weird hair and hands!"*

Sally's mother said she swept her daughter up and ran as fast as she could away from this screaming child. Once she had been returned to the safety of her home, Sally asked, "Mommy, can I have teeth like you and Daddy?"

After enduring all the necessary impressions without even a defiant murmur—much better behavior than most adults exhibit—Sally's "new teeth" were finally ready. The day that I placed her overdentures, I asked if she wanted to see them. She eagerly nodded yes; so I took her by the hand, walked her over to a large mirror, and lifted her up to see her new smile.

Sally didn't say a word. Her face lit up. She smiled—a really, really, really big smile! And, then she blushed!

s a dentist, I consider smiles to be an important and appropriate professional concern. I notice smiles. I keep track of smiles. Of all the smiles I've seen in my life, Sally's was unquestionably the biggest. Sally's smile was the most rewarding thank-you I've ever received. ❤

—Cheryl Lee Willett, DDS, MS

Jane and the Tetracycline Stain

ane was an extremely attractive lady who had been my patient for many years. Her one not-so-attractive feature was her smile—a problem since birth.

When Jane's mother was pregnant, she had been extremely ill and was given large quantities of tetracycline antibiotic. Today, tetracycline is never prescribed during pregnancy because it is known to cause an extremely unattractive, dark-gray, permanent discoloration of the child's adult teeth.

Over the years, Jane and I had often spoken about placing eight beautiful porcelain laminates over her upper front teeth. While this relatively simple procedure would give her a very beautiful smile, it was, unfortunately, very expensive.

One day, Jane walked into my office and announced that because of her son's upcoming marriage, she was finally ready and eager to do the esthetic dentistry.

Treatment progressed rapidly. In just two weeks, her laminates were bonded into place and were absolutely gorgeous. Her new, attractive smile now matched the rest of her appearance. With a promise to return the following morning for a final polishing, Jane rushed out of the office, telling us that she was racing over to her mother's house to show off her new smile.

When Jane returned the next morning, she was sobbing. I

couldn't understand it: Did one of my laminates break? Was she displeased with the results?

To the contrary! On the previous day, when Jane's mother saw her daughter's beautiful new smile, she began crying uncontrollably. Apparently, for all those years, she secretly felt very guilty and blamed herself for taking tetracycline and causing her daughter's unattractive dental condition.

Now that the cosmetic dentistry was completed, all those years of pent-up anguish were released in a torrent of tears. Mother and daughter spent a good part of the night hugging each other and crying in each other's arms.

I found it difficult to control my own emotions as I polished Jane's teeth. I was proud to have been a part of this bittersweet story with a very happy ending. ♥

—Jeffrey M. Galler, DDS, MAGD

Paid in Full

*"Do not withhold good from those who deserve it
when it is in your power to act."*

—Psalms 3:27

 often count the blessings I've received through my career in dentistry—and not all of them have been financial. One blessing is the satisfaction I get from being able to help those less fortunate. While the payment for services may not be monetary, the psychic reward can be tremendous! As a way of identifying deserving patients, I serve as one of many volunteer dentists listed with D-DENT, an agency of the Oklahoma Dental Association dedicated to meeting the dental needs of the poor.

On one occasion, I was called on to provide care for a man pre-qualified by the agency who had no teeth. My new patient—we'll call him Joe to protect his privacy—was a middle-aged man who seemed really nice when I met him. Although I had noticed Joe over a period of several years as he walked up and down the streets of Stillwater, I had never thought much about him before the day he came to my office.

Prior to Joe's first visit, I had been told by a D-DENT case worker that the man needed a full set of dentures. Another volunteer dentist had removed the last of Joe's teeth—they were abscessed—some time earlier, and Joe had been "gumming" it ever since. The caseworker also told me that, since childhood, Joe has not been able to hear or speak—no one knew why. My job was to help Joe eat better than he could without teeth. But I knew communication would be a problem, so I challenged myself to think of ways to deal with the issue. Joe and I really got along well until it came time to take records of his bite relationship. Although he wanted to help me all he could, the process proved just as frustrating for him as it was for me. But since we were both determined to get the job done, persistence and patience prevailed.

Over a period of several weeks, I saw Joe the requisite number of times necessary to prepare a full set of dentures. Finally, the lab work was completed, and they were ready. You could feel it in the air, something was different about that day. The entire staff was on edge—everyone holding their breath in anticipation.

After Joe was seated, I entered the operatory and greeted him. Understandably, he was more than a little anxious—I know I was! Then, just as I had done with so many others before him, I placed the new dentures into my patient's mouth. They fit his gums perfectly! Next, I checked his bite and looked for any overextension of the denture. Everything was fine in that department as well. To wrap things up, I stepped back to look at Joe's profile and noticed that he had put on a big smile. Unfortunately, his handicap prevented him from saying a word.

So far, Joe hadn't seen himself with the dentures—the Moment of Truth had arrived! I handed Joe a mirror, and he studied his new teeth very carefully, as well as taking note of the changes they made in the way his face looked. Then, all of a sudden, his expression changed. His smile was replaced by a frown; he rested the mirror in his lap and turned away. I was puzzled.... Was something wrong?

After a moment, Joe looked at me again. He was crying. And it wasn't long before the entire staff—gathered in the doorway of the operatory—had tears in their eyes. Absolutely nothing was wrong! Joe was overjoyed. Although he couldn't say a word, Joe's face said volumes.

n this life, there are many rewards available to each of us. What we receive from helping our fellow man is right up there near the top. Remind yourself often that much of life has nothing whatsoever to do with money. I don't know what you might think about my experience with Joe, but I believe I was PAID IN FULL! ♥

—J. Walter Coffey, DDS, FAGD, FASDC

2

RAISING SELF-ESTEEM

Once you see a person's
self-image begin to improve,
you will see significant gains
in achievement areas;
but even more important,
you will see a person
who is beginning
to enjoy life more.

—Wayne Dyer

Pat's Final Gift

Every day comes bearing gifts. Untie the ribbons.

—Ann Ruth Schabacker

hen Pat first came into our office, she was already quite sickly, and the advancement of her disease had made her look much older than her forty-eight years. She was thin and drawn, devoid of a smile, and her skin had a gray pallor that made her appear almost ghostlike. Pat was a cancer survivor, but to be honest, it didn't look like she would be surviving much longer. Several years back she had had a total gastrectomy—removal of the stomach. Her required nutrition was gained through a tube that connected to her body and into which a milky liquid was poured. She couldn't eat at all, and when she tried, it made her wretchedly ill.

This nonuse of her teeth and gums had caused Pat some pretty bad dental problems, and by the time she came into the office, she was already missing four lower front teeth. Her previous dentist had replaced these missing teeth with a removable partial denture—the kind of false teeth that clamp to the remaining teeth and are taken out at night. In dentistry, this is not always considered to be the highest level of treatment, but since it was pretty much a foregone conclusion that Pat would be losing her fight with cancer within the next few months, we accepted this removable denture and concentrated on keeping her existing teeth as healthy as possible.

Despite all of this, Pat was a pleasure to be around; and everyone in the office looked forward to her visits. Talking with her, you would never know just how bad her condition was, but as soon as you saw what she looked like, it became obvious that things were on the downhill side of Bad. Nevertheless, she was very proud of her newly found dental health and worked as hard as she could to maintain her regular cleaning appointments and brush and floss on a regular basis.

everal months later, when Pat did not show up for her next cleaning appointment, the office got a collective sinking feeling. No words needed to be said—we all knew what it meant. Trying to reach her relatives proved fruitless, and although a thorough scan of the obituaries for the next few weeks did not turn up her name, we still assumed the worst.

A few weeks had passed when a very strange thing happened—Pat called the office and asked to reschedule her missed cleaning appointment! Now any dental office is used to hearing the world's lamest excuses from patients who miss their cleanings—but can you imagine that Pat was actually apologetic when she explained that her missed appointment was due to a coma?! The hospital doctors had notified her family that she was "on the way out." But there was only one way Pat was leaving that hospital—through the front door!

Her cleaning appointment went well—and she was already back into the routine of taking excellent care of her teeth just several weeks after being comatose. But I was truly shocked when she called me over at the end of her appointment and said, "Dr. Madow, I'd like to consider a more permanent way to replace these missing lower teeth."

Given everything I knew about her failing health and her modest finances, I kind of fumbled around before saying, "Pat, that would be a fantastic way to go in most situations, but we're talking about a pretty big expense here. Normally this would make a lot of sense, but considering your condition, I'm not sure it would be the wisest investment."

To which she replied, "Dr. Madow, you're right. I really don't have much money, and I certainly don't have much time. But I've given this a lot of thought and decided this is the way I want to spend both!"

Well, what else could I say? I explained the procedure, known as an eight-unit bridge, and she made an appointment that day to get started. Several weeks later the treatment was completed and we placed a beautiful fixed bridge on Pat's lower jaw. This treatment is known as "fixed" because the bridge is cemented in place and never leaves the mouth, unlike her previous "removable" denture. Only a dental professional could tell it was there—to everyone else it looked like she had all of her teeth just as Nature intended.

Pat looked the best we had seen her look for quite a while. She was so proud of her new teeth that—for the very first time—she made a tour of the entire office with a huge smile on her face. She gave each of us a big hug and then scheduled her next cleaning.

n the morning of her appointment, we got a phone call from one of Pat's family members explaining that Pat would not be able to make the appointment because she was back in the hospital in another coma. Now, surviving one coma is pretty rare—but the odds against surviving two seemed humungous. Needless to say, we did not try to reschedule the cleaning.

Of course, when you're dealing with someone like Pat, the odds of survival don't mean a whole lot—but we were still shocked when she called the next month—apologizing again and ready to come in for her visit.

When Pat returned, she looked worse than ever before, but she still managed to smile and greet everyone warmly. She never seemed bitter about her illness, and other than the time spent updating her health history, didn't talk about it much at all. As a matter of fact, she never complained much about anything. So I wasn't quite sure what to expect when the hygienist tracked me down in the hallway and said, "Dr. Madow, Pat would like to speak with you about her bridge."

I went into the treatment room and greeted my special patient once again. "Pat, I understand you would like to speak with me about your bridge."

Pat leaned forward and motioned for me to put my ear just a few inches from her mouth. In a barely audible voice, she said, "Dr. Madow, I just want to thank you for this fantastic bridge. It has made such a huge difference in my life."

Seeing the puzzled look on my face, she continued. "You see, I'm not very old, but I realize I don't look all that great. Well, when I was in the hospital with my first coma, I had to take my lower denture out so that they could put that breathing tube down my throat. As I lay in bed, drifting in and out of consciousness, I knew my relatives and friends were in the room visiting me, and there was a good chance that would be the last time they'd ever see me. When I came out of the coma, it really bothered me that their last impression would be of me looking like a toothless old hag. When I got out of the hospital, I made a promise to myself that the same thing would not happen again.

"So this last time, even though I was once again in a coma and had that tube down my throat, at least it was resting against my beautiful new teeth. Just the thought of that made me feel sooooo much younger and prettier.

"So you see, Dr. Madow, by agreeing to do that bridge for me, you gave me a gift that no amount of money can buy. And I just wanted to tell you that in case this is the last time I ever see you."

Well, sadly, that was the last time any of us were to see Pat. But she gave us something that will last forever.

s dentists, even though most of the things we do are fairly routine, every once in a while we are given the privilege to change a life in a very special way, even if that life—like Pat's—is fragile. That is a gift we give that can never be forgotten. And usually, as in this case, the gift returns itself, through us, to everyone we come in contact with.

So Pat, wherever you are, thank you so much for allowing us to give you that gift. We have given it back—in your memory— more times than anyone can count! ♥

—Richard H. Madow, DDS

Gerhardt and Edith

erhardt and Edith came to our office as new patients more than five years ago. Both were in their late sixties at the time. It was immediately clear that Edith was suffering from a form of dementia. Physically, she was a lovely woman, and Gerhardt was proud of her. He was gentle and unfailingly patient as his wife struggled to navigate this life that had come to hold so many unknowns.

Their fiftieth wedding anniversary was coming up soon, and Gerhardt wanted us to do whatever we could to make Edith's teeth look attractive for the celebration. We told him it would require a combination of crowns and veneers—a large investment—but Gerhardt didn't hesitate to accept the plan. When the procedures on his wife were complete, he was delighted. The stress of his wife's dementia meant that her smile was more infrequent and hesitant than it had been when she was younger, but it was once again as beautiful as the rest of her. Even Edith seemed pleased.

The couple had a small family celebration after which Gerhardt took Edith on a wonderful European tour. Shortly before they left, she had started taking a new medication that seemed to restore some memory and peace, so she enjoyed the trip immensely. They came home with high hopes for the future, but her improvement was short-lived. Within months she was again consumed by dementia.

Edith rarely slept and could not be still. Gerhardt was constantly exhausted and beside himself with grief. After consulting with the Mayo Clinic, he was forced to find an extended-care facility for his wife. For the first time in 50 years, they were not together. Daily he would visit her, help to dress and feed her, and take her for rides in the car—the only place she could really relax. But ultimately, anxiety and restlessness took their toll on her body and, after some months, she died.

At his dental visit immediately following Edith's death, Gerhardt shared with us the details of her final months. His voice trembled as he spoke. The doctor and I found ourselves wiping away tears as he told us how much he loved her and how lonesome he was.

But at one point during the story, Gerhardt's face lit up and he smiled. He was anxious for us to know that when Edith was admitted to the extended-care facility, a nurse commented on her teeth. She asked if they were really Edith's own teeth. Gerhardt's voice seemed stronger as he told us how proud he was to be able to say they were. The nurse's comment was "Why, she's many years older than I am, but her teeth are so much more beautiful!" He seemed to understand our discomfort with the idea that after such a large investment, Edith couldn't enjoy her new smile for a longer period. He let us know that even if he had known how little time she had, he would have made the same decision. It was the nicest expression of appreciation we could have ever asked.

erhardt and Edith have taught us valuable lessons. At a time in life when the body could no longer be counted on to serve as it used to, the knowledge that their teeth were their own gave them a source of pride and dignity. They are role models for our lives and reason enough to be involved in this wonderful profession of dentistry. ♥

—Sue O'Brien, RDH

Never Too Late

What greater thing is there for two human souls
than to feel that they are joined for life—
to strengthen each other in all labor,
to rest on each other in all sorrow,
to minister to each other in all pain,
to be one with each other in silent,
unspeakable memories at
the moment of the last parting?

—George Eliot

ne of the most charming dental patients I have ever met came to my office with her husband and wanted only an upper denture. They were both in their late sixties. She was plainly dressed and wore no makeup. He was tall with a comfortable bearing. He didn't say much, except to inquire about the cost.

I assumed my new patient wanted a replacement denture, so I asked her what teeth she was wearing now. She said she had grown up in a North Carolina mountain town and had lost her teeth in her twenties. She had been without teeth for 40 years!

I asked about her diet—what she could or could not eat. She told me she ate whatever she pleased—corn on the cob, apples, spare ribs, chicken...you name it. She said she didn't need the new teeth to eat; it was her husband who wanted her to have them so that she wouldn't feel "old."

n the day that I delivered her top denture, the couple was right on time for her appointment. He wore a starched dress shirt buttoned to the collar with no tie; and she wore a pretty straw hat, flowered cotton dress, and white gloves.

When the deliver-and-comfort checks on her denture were finished, her husband came into the business office and paid with $100 bills. He looked at his wife and told her how nice her new teeth looked, extended his arm for her to hold, and walked out the door.

She turned around and shyly said, "It's our 50th wedding anniversary today." ♥

—A.T. Williams, DDS

The Hidden Smile

You have not lived a perfect day,
even though you have earned your money,
unless you have done something for someone
who will never be able to repay you.

—Ruth Smeltzer

hen I met our new patient, Connie, I had been a dental assistant for just over a year and was still learning the basics. We established an immediate rapport and visited for quite a while during her appointment. She shared with me some of the heartache—as well as the happy moments—of her career as a counselor of troubled families. In turn, I shared a few of my own learning experiences—some which made me laugh and others that made me cry.

Connie then started to say something when she caught herself and suddenly stopped. Wanting her to feel comfortable, I gently asked that she tell me what was on her mind. Although it appeared difficult for her to continue, she paused a moment and then asked, "Jackie, have you ever wanted to help someone but weren't able to—financially or physically—and couldn't stop thinking about it?"

She then told me of a boy, Michael, and his parents that she had been counseling. Michael was handsome and doing very well in school; but he seemed ill at ease every time she spoke with him. And he never smiled! One day his mother confided that Michael was self-conscious about his bad teeth. His parents were unable to take him to the dentist because they had lost their insurance and his mother was certain her son had cavities because of the black spots on his teeth.

Connie sat quietly for a few moments but finally found the courage to ask if the dentist, Dr. Lais, would consider helping this young man. She spoke so quickly I could hardly get a word in edgewise, assuring me that she would provide Michael's transportation and pay as much as she could for his treatment—whenever she could. I knew that Connie had her own family to support and that what she was proposing would be a great sacrifice for her. I promised I would discuss the situation with the dentist right away.

As I left the room, I started to get excited at the prospect of Connie's being able to tell this young man she could help him. I approached Dr. Lais during his first free moment and explained the situation. He promised he would talk with Connie before she left the office. I wasn't sure what he was going to say, but I still felt very excited.

When Dr. Lais entered the room, Connie and I were both sick with anticipation. She told the dentist she would understand if he felt she was asking too much but would appreciate it if he'd at least consider looking at the boy. Dr. Lais agreed to do so and asked that she set up an examination appointment.

At last the day came for Michael's exam. With a mixture of pride and protectiveness, Connie escorted the handsome-but-shy young man into the office and introduced him to Dr. Lais and me. Although we smiled and greeted him with warm enthusiasm, Michael kept his head down and stared at the floor. Embarrassment over his smile was definitely affecting his social skills!

As Dr. Lais proceeded with the examination, I soon realized that Michael would need extensive treatment. We took X rays and photographs and explained to both the patient and to Connie the treatment he would need. She was anxious and wanted to know when we could get started. She also told Dr. Lais that she and her husband had decided to put Michael's bill on their charge card. We rearranged the schedule for the day and began treatment immediately.

Michael was silent throughout the entire appointment. Dr. Lais and I worked very hard at removing decay and placing composite restorations on all of Michael's front teeth. He seemed to be handling the extensive treatment quite well.

Finally, after a few hours, Dr. Lais pulled away from the chair and asked Connie to take a look. When she saw the numb smile on Michael's face, she burst out in a mild scream. She turned to Dr. Lais and gave him a big hug before instructing Michael to stand up and look in the wall mirror.

The boy seemed shocked at what he saw. The smile that had been hiding for all those years was finally revealed. He grabbed Connie and gave her a huge hug and kept whispering, "Thank you so much, thank you."

Dr. Lais told Michael, "Young man, you have a whole lot to thank Connie for; I hope your new smile makes life a little easier!"

Michael held out his hand for Dr. Lais to shake. The dentist took it and pulled Michael in for a big hug. Dr. Lais then turned to Connie and said, "I'm going to put a smile on your face too—there is no charge for the treatment." Connie responded with instant tears of relief that quickly gave way— as Dr. Lais had anticipated—to another huge smile.

hat an experience—to feel that much joy for someone else! Every day when I get up in the morning, I can't help but think about all those people who have so much to be happy about but who have yet to reveal their hidden smile. ♥

—Jackie Lais, CDA, CDPMA

A Good Boy

To feel loved, to belong,
to have a place and to hear
one's dignity and worth often affirmed—
these are to the soul
what food is to the body.

—Anne Ortlund

 y new patient was a five-year-old named Danny, scheduled that morning for his first-ever dental appointment. And according to Cathy, my recep-tionist, he was squeezed into the schedule on an emergency basis.

Danny lived with his grandparents—a couple in their late seventies—who at this very late stage in their lives were raising their little grandson. Their own son, Danny's dad, was in San Quentin Prison, and his mother's whereabouts were unknown since she had deserted her family two years earlier.

Now before I go any further, I should explain that I am a specialist in pediatric dentistry and as such, frequently have "difficult" children referred to my practice by area dentists. Danny was such a patient. In our office, my staff and I take great satisfaction in being able to "turn around" these children and make them into good patients for succeeding dental and medical appointments. Furthermore, it has always been our unvarying custom—it's really a *rule* in our office—that no little patient, no matter how he or she has behaved during an appointment, ever leaves without being congratulated for something, even if it's only for being "the best 'spitter' we've had all day!"

You get the idea.

When his turn came, Danny had to be brought into the operatory a bit forcibly by one of my dental assistants. Of course this is not an unusual behavior for children, especially children of that age, on their first-ever dental appointment. Danny's grandmother let us know she was quite worried that he might misbehave.

After a few brief minutes of explanation—with a reassuring arm around his shoulder as we talked—Danny soon quieted down and took a great interest in watching the procedures in the mirror I had handed him. In no time at all, I completed the emergency treatment and invited his grandmother back into the operatory to explain what I had done. Meanwhile, Danny picked out his little gift from our toy drawer since every child who visits our practice receives a gift upon leaving—regardless of how they behave.

 week later, a full 15 minutes before he was even due for his follow-up appointment, the door to the operatory burst open and Danny tore into the room eager to be seated in the chair. This was also not an unusual event for children in our practice.

This appointment went even better than Danny's first, and Grandma came back into the operatory once again. And once again, she was profuse in expressing her pleasure with Danny's acceptance of dental treatment.

"All week long, Danny has asked me several times a day when he was going to be taken back to the dentist. And do you know why Danny was so anxious to return?" Grandma asked.

"No," I responded. "Please tell us."

"Because you told him he was a good boy."

Here was an emotionally hurting little five-year-old who

had never been told—before that first visit—that he was a "good boy." How very sad. But how much joy and reinforcement Grandma's comment has given my staff and me over the succeeding years. ❤

—Robert C. Smithwick, DDS, FACD

Sammy

everal years ago, a young girl came to our office looking for a fourth opinion. The previous three dentists she had seen wanted to extract all of her teeth and give her full, removable dentures. She seemed very nervous about the visit. I looked at her chart expecting to see 13 or 14 written in the age box. To my shock and surprise, I learned she was 19 years old! I looked back at her face and concluded she must be anorexic. Her shoulders were slumped forward; and, as she stared at her feet, her thin, unkempt blond hair fell in front of her face.

After introductions, I learned that my new patient's name was Samantha. She told me she suffered from an unusual birth defect in that most of her "permanent" teeth never came in. Her mouth was largely populated with a variety of "baby" teeth, most of them loose. In fact, some teeth were so loose they would have flown out with a good hard sneeze. Two of the front teeth were barely hanging on by a flap of skin. The only opposing teeth that touched were the two upper and two lower front teeth that dentists call "centrals."

When she ate, Sammy had to cut everything into the smallest possible pieces, slicing meat as small as a dime. She had to chew everything on those rabbit-like front teeth. She preferred to take her food as a liquid or in soft form such as omelets, oatmeal, milkshakes, or yogurt. The idea of biting into a sandwich was horrifying to her because she could lose half her remaining teeth. A hamburger was out of the question. Salads, candy bars, steaks, cookies, bread, and popcorn were unthinkable. The only way this girl could eat vegetables was with the help of a blender.

Sammy regularly turned down invitations to lunch with friends or coworkers because she was so self-conscious of her eating habits. Dating was difficult because guys always wanted to take her to nice restaurants where she would have to crumble the bread into tiny balls in order to eat. She was afraid to kiss because the loose front teeth might come out and cause her— and her date—huge embarrassment. Sammy's teeth were causing great trouble in her social life. Her coworkers all thought she was stuck up, and the men asking for dinner dates were rejected immediately without knowing why.

Sammy was ashamed of her condition and didn't want anyone to know why she appeared to be so antisocial. Instead she retreated into her little cocoon—feeling sorry for herself and rejecting everyone around her. This in turn caused others to ignore or reject her. The isolation from society caused Sammy to doubt her self worth and resulted in low self-esteem.

Through my dental assistant, I learned a great deal more about our newest patient. (It's quite common in the dental field that patients will be formal with their dentist but will warm up to a friendly dental assistant. My assistant is quite chatty and quickly puts people at ease.)

We learned that Sammy had a low-paying, dead-end job as well as an abusive boyfriend. She was terrified of eating and only picked at food like a bird. Her poor nutrition resulted in frequent illness. Because of her teeth, Sammy's social life and her health were a mess.

After careful study of her dentition, we were able to conclude that Sammy had enough permanent teeth to make "roundhouses" on both her upper and lower arches. This is permanent bridge-work that goes around the entire arch and is anchored in the mouth. The previous three dentists wanted to pull everything and make removable dentures. The idea of losing all of her teeth and having full dentures was horrifying to 19-year-old Sammy because she envisioned her face all collapsed in, with wrinkles, making her look like an old lady. The fact that we recommended restoration of her mouth with a solid set of fully functional and esthetic teeth gave her tremendous hope and lifted her spirits.

Sammy, from whose mouth we were going to remove most of the remaining teeth, was an emotional wreck at first. It took a lot of handholding and several visits devoted exclusively to discussion before we could begin actual procedures. We arranged it so that she would always have some type of temporary bridge in her mouth and never had to walk around with spaces showing. Fortunately, we have a dental laboratory in our building so the technician can work closely with our team.

As her treatment progressed, Sammy became quite interested in the details of the lab work and we spent many hours making small changes. I always scheduled her for several hours before the end of the day so we could take our time. I'd make one small change and then let her examine the results for ten minutes while I worked on someone else. She looked at her crowns in a mirror and picked at each minute detail. I'd make another small change and then let her inspect the latest version for another ten minutes.

Each of these visits took an average of two to three hours. While this process strained the patience of our staff—and the technician cringed every time he heard Sammy's name—I was pleased that she wanted to take an active role in her own treatment.

When Sammy finally got her new solid set of teeth, she was initially afraid to chew with them—old habits die hard. Continuing to eat like a bird, it took a good six months before she was comfortable chewing semisolid food—and another six months after that before she attempted to chew vigorously. Today, Sammy can—and does—eat anything she wants.

It didn't take long before Sammy's emaciated frame started to fill in. Although she's still slender, she now radiates a vibrant, healthy glow. With better nutrition—she regularly eats fruits and vegetables—Sammy isn't sick nearly as often. Almost immediately, she started to regain her confidence. She got a better job with career prospects and dumped the abusive boyfriend. Eating in restaurants with coworkers and going out on dates was suddenly possible.

As her self-esteem improved, Sammy started dressing better, had her hair done, began exercising, corrected her posture, and took better care of herself. She is now a beautiful and talented woman with high self-esteem. Today, Sammy is working her way up the career ladder and has married a very nice man—a fellow corporate executive.

ammy's case illustrates how important proper nutrition and self-esteem can be to our overall wellbeing. Every week, we see people at our office who are down on their luck. They want just one tooth pulled—and then they're gone until the next time something hurts. Their lives get just a little bit worse with each tooth they lose. These people feel they're trapped in that lifestyle and use money as an excuse. They fail to appreciate that America really is the land of opportunity where success is a matter of character and initiative.

While my staff and I would like to take credit for turning Sammy's life around, in reality it was she who pulled herself up by the bootstraps. We simply helped her attain the goals she set for herself. Having seen the transformation Sammy was able to achieve on her own initiative, I'm convinced anyone else with enough determination can do the same. ❤

—D. Michael Hart, DDS, FAGD, MAGD

Sheila's Diastema

heila was a lovely 21-year-old, and a member of a large family of loyal patients. For years, I had urged her and her parents to let me fix the large, unpleasant-looking gap (diastema) between her two front teeth. Suddenly, late on a Thursday afternoon, Sheila called and begged the receptionist to give her an emergency appointment. We had no choice but to offer to stay late and schedule her in the early evening.

When I greeted Sheila, I was pretty tired; it had been a long day. "What's the emergency?" I asked, "How can I help you?"

The patient explained that it was suddenly imperative to have her gap-toothed smile bonded immediately—right then and there.

"But, Sheila," I protested, "we've discussed this for years. Cosmetic bonding isn't exactly an emergency problem."

She explained, respectfully and apologetically, that she had a blind date for Saturday night; that all her friends assured her that this guy was the man of her dreams; and, that she wanted to look her very best for this momentous occasion. Before she even completed her explanation, my assistants already realized that I—ever the romantic—couldn't help but honor Sheila's request. One hour later, the job was done, and a beautiful, perfectly aligned, glistening smile appeared.

Several months later, Sheila showed up at the office bursting with excitement. "I'm engaged to David, that blind date," she exclaimed, "and it's all thanks to you!"

I accepted her compliment in my usual, humble fashion and explained that she had always looked beautiful, and that perhaps the bonding merely gave her a little extra self-confidence.

"No, Doctor, you don't understand," she gushed. "After David proposed to me, and I, of course, accepted, I asked him a certain question." Sheila explained that she somehow got the courage to ask her new fiancé a question that had been bothering her. It seems that on their first few dates, he constantly stared at her teeth.

I asked, "Really? What did he say?"

Sheila continued her story. Her fiancé confessed that all his friends had told him Sheila would be his perfect soulmate, but that she had one bad feature: an ugly space between her two front teeth.

He told her, "On our first dates, I kept staring at your teeth, looking for that space. I couldn't find it. Instead, I fell in love with your beautiful smile." ❤

—Jeffrey M. Galler, DDS, MAGD

Teeth Maketh the Man

An old man in love is like a flower in winter.

—English Proverb

've known Henry for years. We met when my family lived in south Georgia. Henry and I shared a passion for making model airplanes and flying them in free-flight competition. He was a fixture at the meetings. You would see him in Georgia, Tennessee, and North Carolina, flying his beautiful creations and winning the "Over-70's Free-Flight Competition" four years in a row.

Everyone knew Henry. It wouldn't be a meeting if we didn't see him chasing a plane across a field, his sandy hair flying in the breeze, his tall, thin figure running fast for a man his age. Henry was the retired farmer with the toothless grin.

"Why don't you make Henry some teeth?" someone asked me one day. "You're a dentist. Couldn't you fix him up?"

"Yes, I'll do it," I promised. I waved at Henry and motioned him to stroll on over to where I was standing. "Come and see me in Monroe sometime. I'll make you some teeth, and it won't cost you anything."

Ten days later, Henry showed up at the office for impressions. About a week after that, I had his dentures ready. They made a huge improvement in the old man's appearance. It gave me a great feeling when he drove away in his truck, waving and flashing those gleaming new pearly whites at me.

Henry missed the next two competitions; and it was about a year before I saw him again. There he was, standing at the edge of the field, tall and straight, the sandy hair neatly cut, his weathered face split in a wide smile. The teeth made him look ten years younger. There was something else about him, too. He looked excited and happy; and he smiled and smiled and smiled."Are you flying in this round, Henry?" I asked.

"Nope. Don't do that no more. I'm done with flying. Ain't got time for model airplanes.... See that pretty woman over there? She don't look 60, does she?"

"She's very attractive, Henry. But how come you're not in the over-70 competition? Are you staying out this year so that someone else can have a chance at winning?"

"Nope. I'm staying out because I'm done with it. That woman over there likes me. She likes the way I smile. We do everything together. She don't build model airplanes. See, Doc, I ain't got time for model airplanes, and I ain't got time for any of you—now that I got me some teeth." ♥

—Kenneth Grubbs, DDS

Temp Rewards

All people smile in the same language.

—Anonymous

fter learning I was pregnant with our first child, I decided to seek employment as a dental hygiene "temp" in addition to my regular four-day-a-week job as a hygienist in another practice. Since "blessed events" can place an unexpected financial burden on parents-to-be, my husband and I felt it would be wise to supplement our modest savings in this way.

Soon after I arrived at the office of my part-time employer, I met Marino, the assistant who would be helping me whenever he could. His contribution to my efforts would prove invaluable. Even though I took him away from his normal routine, he was willing to help at any time without complaint, always maintaining a pleasant smile and a great attitude! With his help, everything fell into place, and my first day began to brighten and become less stressful.

When I went to the reception area to bring back my third patient, Maria, I became uneasy. Although her eyeliner, makeup, and clothing were perfect—including her matching navy hat—she seemed resolute and unsmiling as I introduced myself and led her back to my room. Her chart indicated it had been two years since her last visit; and as I started to update her medical history, she stared at me blankly. Finally, with confusion evident in the tone of her voice, she responded in Spanish. Since I don't speak that language, I realized we could not communicate; and this put an uncomfortable wedge between us. I held up my index finger and gestured for Maria to wait a moment. I then tracked down Marino and asked, "Do you, by any chance, speak Spanish?"

With a smile and a wink, he responded, *"Sí, Señora."*

I was saved again as he followed me into the operatory, now to be my interpreter. Together, we updated Maria's health history and medications and discovered that she had just ended her second bout of chemotherapy and radiation treatments for cancer. At that point, I realized why she wore the navy blue hat—she had no hair. When I finally examined her mouth, I further understood why she didn't smile. Due to the medications she had taken and the treatments she had undergone, her entire dentition was coated with an ugly brown-to-black stain. Knowing that her dental treatment would take a while, I checked the clock. Fortunately, my mask covered my frown. Updating the health history had taken more time than I had planned, and I now had just 30 minutes remaining before my next patient was due.

As I began to scale Maria's teeth, I accepted the fact there was no way I could complete her procedure in the scheduled time. I then decided to simply forget about the clock. My concern shifted to making this patient feel really good about herself. Maria proved to be a "patient" patient and was easy to work with. When I was finally satisfied that all of the stains had been removed to the best of my ability, I raised her chair in preparation for the doctor's exam. Again with no conversation, only hand gestures, I tried to let her know why we were waiting.

After an awkward few minutes, I decided to offer the patient a mirror to let her see the results of my efforts but couldn't find one in the unfamiliar office. Once again Marino came to my rescue, locating a mirror and holding it up for her.

I stood behind Maria and could see her reflected face as she looked at her teeth. My emotions heightened, and a warm feeling gushed through me when she first smiled. She quickly covered her mouth with her hand—as though in disbelief—and then pulled her hand away slowly and smiled again. As I watched, Maria's entire face emitted this warm, bright ray of sunshine that filled the entire room. She absolutely shrieked with joy. She then turned to Marino and began speaking excitedly while at the same time smiling and crying because she was so happy.

he next thing I knew, Maria jumped out of the dental chair and hugged me. Although I couldn't speak Spanish, and she couldn't speak English, we both communicated in that universal language—tears of joy. We understood each other perfectly. She told Marino she had not seen the "natural" color of her teeth in years. Maria was ecstatic with the knowledge that she could once again face the world with a smile.

She told us that due to the cancer treatments, she had lost all of her hair—including her eyebrows and eyelashes. (She had even had these areas tattooed—no wonder her eyeliner was so perfect!) I had never known anyone who did this; and through Marino we discussed the time and pain it took for her to accomplish this makeover. She said it didn't matter what she had to endure, just so long as she could look like a normal person and not a "cancer patient."

The huge hug Maria gave me, the smile she displayed for the doctor as he examined her teeth, the smile she gave to the receptionist, and the smile she wore as she left the office uplifted my heart! Maybe it was my pregnancy hormones that made me feel such a deep emotional connection with Maria, or maybe it was just seeing the true goodness, sincerity, and gratitude she expressed so freely. Whatever it was, I was elated to have been a part of this happening and to experience that wonderful warm feeling that rushed through my body—from my head all the way to my toes. I have no doubt my unborn child also shared in the special glow of that day. ❤

—Karen L. Hart-Sabol, RDH

I Feel Rich!

Treat people as if they are what they ought to be,
and you help them become what they are capable of being.

—Johann W. van Goethe (1749-1832)

ven though our practice is located in a moderately affluent Memphis suburb, we still treat a few Medicaid and indigent patients. Lashanta was such a person—13 years old, extremely poor, and on welfare. Her hair was matted, her clothes were unkempt and ill-fitting, she lived in the decaying Housing Authority projects, and she rode a bus to the office because her family had no car. You just knew by looking that her cleanliness and oral hygiene left something to be desired. She was one of the desperate, neglected kids the inner city breeds and discards without a second thought.

In our office, Lashanta was not treated differently than any other patient. But how were we to know what sort of impression we were making on her? As with every patient, we showered her with soft, gentle voices; we delivered compassionate smiles; and we talked about standards and values—character development and what it has to do with the direction one takes in life.

During her third filling appointment, Lashanta looked up at me and said, "I love coming here."

We all know it's unusual to hear that from any dental

patient, let alone a 13-year-old girl who would probably rather be talking with friends on the phone or chasing boys. My response was, "That's nice. Why do you like coming here?"

" 'Cause you all make me feel rich!" she answered.

WOW! What a penetrating statement. There I stood, dressed in my polo shirt, looking at her with frightened horse eyes and freshly scrubbed youthful ignorance. Lashanta had pierced me to the core; she had connected—and left me with a powerful lesson about people's feelings.

I learned that it makes no difference whether your patients are rich or poor—black, white, yellow, red, or green—they all want to be loved, appreciated, and made to feel they have value. We had treated Lashanta just like every other patient, but—to her—it was acceptance into a world she wasn't accustomed to. If we had given her a look of disgust and dismissal—what most people direct to the less fortunate, she would have dug deeper into her shell. To her, the reception she received from us was far beyond what she had ever expected. As a result, she felt as though she was our favorite patient—and she had become just that! We raised her self-esteem. In return, she renewed our sense of purpose and reinforced our philosophy about treating all patients with the same courtesy and care.

 have no idea what Lashanta is doing now; but I can only hope the feelings of self-worth we gave her were encouragement enough for her to raise herself to a higher socioeconomic level. I'd like to believe she left our practice believing she was rich—special, unique, rare—and that there was no other child like her in the whole world. She certainly made us believe in her; she made a real difference in our lives! Thank you, Lashanta. ♥

—Donald L. Gary, DDS

Credit Report

There's right, and there's wrong.
You get to do one or the other.
You do one, and you're living.
You do the other,
and you may be walking around,
but you're as dead as a beaver hat.

—John Wayne

s the administrator of our dental office, part of my job is to make sure the practice is paid in full for professional services rendered. Occasionally, we have patients who promise to pay—cross their hearts and hope to die—but do not. When we hear the phrases, "I forgot my checkbook," or "Just bill me," our experience always makes us wonder if we will ever be paid.

One day, I had a lady call who said she was down on her luck, had a terrible toothache, and needed a root canal—not an inexpensive procedure. But she was temporarily broke, she told me. She explained that she was a single mother of three, her previous employer had recently laid her off, and she had just found a new job. She promised she would make a payment every month and send more when she could. She seemed like a genuinely nice person on the phone, but I worried about extending her credit. Finally, I realized that I had a really good feeling about her. I was especially impressed that she was so honest up front.

We did the root canal on Miss Virginia; and every month she sent me her payment. Some months she would send a little more. But one day she walked into my office with a red face and her head down. I could tell something was wrong. She told me her sister had taken ill and she felt she had to visit her. She said she would feel better if she had the extra money—that month's scheduled payment—with her.

She told me she would understand if we could not allow her to lapse on a payment. She also said she knew we had made a big exception in allowing her to pay over time and did not want to let us down.

I assured our patient it would not be a problem—that she had proven her credit was good. I wished her sister well—and her, a safe trip home. After she left, I couldn't help but feel overwhelmed at the character she had shown. So, in spite of my hectic schedule, I took time to write her a note:

Dear Miss Virginia,

I had to drop you a line to tell you what a fine person you are. Please know that we understand your situation and hope that, in time, things will become easier for you. We have enjoyed having you as a patient as well as meeting such a genuinely good person. Our thoughts and prayers are with you.

Keep well, and may God be with you and yours always.

Sincerely,
Amy McLamb

I really didn't expect a response. But a month later, the patient was in my office again. This time, her face was bright and her head was held high. She had my note in her hand.

She told me that no one—ever in her life—had said those things to her. Since she was a child, she had been told she was worthless and sorry. She said my kind words meant a lot to her and that she would keep my note forever. She then handed me her last check with a smile and a tear.

hinking back on that experience, I realize I almost didn't take time to write this nice lady. I'm so glad I did! After she left the office, I wrote another note—this time to my parents—thanking them for always being positive with me and giving me their support. ♥

—Amy M. McLamb

3

COMPASSION AND KINDNESS

*If you have no charity,
you have the worst kind
of heart trouble.*

—Bob Hope

The Farnham Legacy

"Once you find the way, you'll be bound.
It will obsess you, but believe me,
it will be a magnificent obsession."

—Lloyd C. Douglas

 was a married dental student in the early eighties with an infant daughter. We moved from the West to the Midwest so that I could attend school. We had no family in the area and lived a distance from the school. Making ends meet with a limited income was a challenge, and setting aside money with which to cover medical expenses was almost impossible.

Then our daughter became ill. She had four ear infections in as many months. It cost about $25 to take her to the doctor and buy her Amoxicillin antibiotic for each episode. A couple of times we used money we had received from our parents for a special occasion to cover these expenses.

While I was conversing with a fellow dental student about my problems, he told me of a local pediatrician who treated the children of dental students at no charge and gave me the doctor's phone number. This wonderful man, Dr. Paul Farnham, Jr., took care of our daughter and also a second daughter born two years later.

That semester, I learned of a fellow dental student whose daughter had contracted bronchitis and required immediate medical treatment in order to avoid the risk of pneumonia. He called Dr. Farnham on a Saturday evening. Even though the doctor had been on his way to the symphony, he came into the office and treated the little girl. When my friend offered to pay him, the payment was refused. Instead Dr. Farnham suggested that in the future my friend could do the same for someone else.

r. Farnham died suddenly during my third year of dental school. It was at his funeral that the reason for his kindness was revealed. His own father, Dr. Paul Farnham, Sr., had been a married dental student with children, and a kind doctor had provided free medical care for his family during his school years. The only thing the other doctor asked was that someday he could help someone else as he had been helped.

I am sure the younger Dr. Farnham repaid the kindness shown his father a hundredfold by caring for the children of dental students for many years. We have always remembered him and try to continue his wonderful legacy. ❤

—Bert F. Engstrom, DMD

Full Circle

The game of life is the game of boomerangs.
Our thoughts, words, and deeds
return to us—sooner or later—
with astounding accuracy.

—Florence Shinn

t was a typical day in our endodontic office where we perform root canal and other specialized dental procedures. I was attending to the normally scheduled patients as well as numerous "up all night" emergencies. After anesthetizing Denise, my patient in Room 4, I proceeded to the adjacent operatory a few short steps away to assess an emergency patient who had just arrived.

Stephanie was in her late forties and spoke very little English. Fortunately, her sister-in-law accompanied her as a translator. After a brief introduction, I learned Stephanie had arrived in this country only a few months earlier and had been up all night with excruciating pain.

When it was explained that an X ray would be needed so that I could determine an appropriate treatment, a look of worry came over her face. You see, Stephanie did not have insurance, and finances were a real and troubling concern for her. Working as a cook, Stephanie was saving her modest income to make arrangements for her entire family to come to America. As the two discussed financial considerations, I excused myself to return to Room 4 and finish the treatment on Denise.

When I came back to Stephanie's room, the discussion seemed quite far from a resolution. At that point, seeing Stephanie's dilemma, I offered to do the consultation at no charge. They were very appreciative, and I instructed my assistant to proceed with the X ray.

Denise had apparently overheard some of my conversation with Stephanie. As she got up from the dental chair to leave, Denise stated that she would like to pay for the treatment of the woman in the next room because "finances shouldn't prevent her from getting the best care available." I commented that this gesture was very kind, but I was already doing the consultation at no charge.

Denise then clarified her intentions. She indicated she wanted to pay for the entire root canal procedure as well as the crown that would be required after the treatment.

I was astonished. Denise stated that the only stipulation was that she remain completely anonymous. I asked Denise to wait a moment so I could diagnose Stephanie's situation— and collect my thoughts.

Stephanie, indeed, needed a root canal but was otherwise in very good dental health. I relayed the diagnosis and treatment plan to Denise, and on her way out, she left a check for the full amount to pay for Stephanie's procedure. Additionally, she asked who Stephanie's general dentist was so that she could contact the office to pay for the crown.

When I relayed the news to Stephanie and her sister-in-law, there were tears of joy and amazement. Stephanie's sister-in-law mentioned that Stephanie had spent much of her adult life doing charitable work and helping others—now it had come full circle.

ven on our most routine days, the presence of the Divine can break through and make us take pause. Denise and I talked a bit, and she shared a phrase that will always remain with me: "I have come to

realize it is far better to be able to give than to *have* to receive."
I feel fortunate to have met Denise and been a vehicle for this
wondrous act of kindness. ❤

—Lisa M. Wendell, DMD

One Winter

udy's 90-year-old mother, Esther, had fallen and broken her hip. During her hospital stay, Esther's upper false teeth had been lost. On a snowy December morning, Judy telephoned our office manager, Adrienne, and inquired, "Does the dentist make house calls?"

That winter was the worst on record—14 snowstorms in all. Although our office is wheelchair accessible, all the snow made it impossible for Esther to come in. Frail and weak from her hospital stay, the old woman was withering away since she could not eat properly without her teeth.

Adrienne listened carefully as Judy described the problem and provided the necessary information for me to decide on a course of action. Adrienne promised to get back to Judy by the end of the day. The request for a house call was something new for me. Although I had never made one before, I was willing to study the details to see if it would be possible.

I sat down and thought about Esther. Could I possibly be of help? In my mind, I began to develop a step-by-step plan to make her a full upper denture. For the proper preparation of such an appliance, five appointments are required, plus one or two additional visits for adjustments. Certainly the technical aspects of a home visit could be accomplished. Material for impressions can be mixed anywhere; I could use a small butane torch for setting the teeth and recording a bite; and I had a portable electric lathe that would be perfect for the inevitable adjustments. Adrienne called Judy to arrange the consultation visit at Esther's home.

It was cold and snowing the day Adrienne and I stopped by. Esther's live-in aide, Dolly, opened the door and led us into the warm kitchen where Judy greeted us. Esther sat quietly by the stove, slumped in her wheelchair. The old woman looked extremely thin and frail; but that didn't interfere with her hospitality. As soon as the introductions were completed, she offered us a platter of Dolly's homemade chocolate chip cookies. She also explained that she couldn't eat any herself because the chips were too hard for her gums. While Esther spoke, she held a hand over her mouth to obscure the fact she had no teeth.

I continued the conversation by saying, "It's nice to meet you all…especially you, Esther. You're lucky to have a daughter like Judy; she's very concerned for you. Now let me explain how we're going to make your new teeth right here in the kitchen."

Judy had a few questions: "Will it hurt my mom? How many visits will the process take? Can I be of any help?"

Adrienne and I reassured everyone there would be little or no discomfort.

I asked Esther if she was prepared to see me twice a week.

"Heck, yes!" she shouted, "Every day, if you like."

We all laughed, and I got started on making the preliminary impression then and there.

Adrienne and I made two house calls each week—on Monday and Thursday—working through our office lunch hour to help Esther. My lab was very responsive and expedited every step in the case. It was a joy to watch Esther perk up a bit more each time we visited. Finally, the day came to deliver her new teeth.

No longer slumped down, Esther demonstrated her best wheelchair posture, back ramrod straight with hands folded in her lap, while I fitted the new teeth. Judy and Dolly were very pleased with Esther's new smile. "They look so natural," commented her daughter.

Esther chimed in, "Where are those chocolate chip cookies? I've been dying to have some ever since I got back from the hospital."

After that, I returned to the house two more times for adjustments. With her new denture, Esther looked like a different person. She became perky, loved to chitchat and, when she spoke, her hand no longer covered her mouth.

When spring rolled around, the office received a lovely letter from Judy. Adrienne opened it and left the message on my desk.

Dear Dr. Novick and Adrienne,

I have always been afraid of going to the dentist. Well, all doctors really, but especially the dentist. My mom always brought us there when we were kids because she did not want us to lose our teeth the way she had.

My mom really liked you, Doctor Novick. She said you were kind to her. She could tell that you really cared, and that you were a patient man.

My mom passed away recently, but she loved those teeth you made for her. She always said that, thanks to you, she could eat well. Your kindness and hard work gave her a better quality of life for her last months.

Thank you,
Judy

I put the letter down and made a mental note to send Judy a card. A part of me felt sad, while some other part felt really good. It was—and continues to be—a blessing to know that a dentist can make a difference in the world by helping just one person. ♥

—Steven Novick, DDS

Steak for the Colonel

'm a small-town dentist with mobile dental equipment, and on occasion, I treat patients at long-term care facilities, hospitals, or private homes. John Howard is a retired Army officer from WWII subsisting on a small pension with his foreign-born wife, Annie. For the last two years, he has been homebound due to bouts with emphysema complicated by adult onset diabetes. Annie called my office late one afternoon and, in a heavy accent, asked if I could treat her husband in their home. She explained that he had "broken his plate." I assured her I would stop by the next day and bring my equipment with me.

After receiving the Howards' address, I realized they lived in a neighborhood I had never been to before. I was sure this section of town had not seen many dentists, especially carrying their equipment in tow. The area had a bad reputation. That, and a visit scheduled at the end of the day, put me in a gloomy mood for my drive to their apartment.

As I neared my destination, I realized I might have my hands full. Graffiti covered the buildings, trash was all over the grounds, and many buildings had no number on the outside. After driving around and around the parking lots, seeking directions was in order.

Several teenagers were standing on the corner, and I asked if they knew where the Howards lived. The answer came quickly, was not the least bit helpful, and couldn't be repeated here for reasons I'll leave to your imagination.

After another lap, I was able to guess at the missing numbers on the buildings and found my destination. Annie stood at the door waiting impatiently. She demanded to know why I was late. The directness with which she asked was made more pointed by her broken English. This was not the recommended way to start a professional association, and we were both disappointed.

Next, she escorted me to her living room. The odor of medicine and the constant put-put-put sound of a humidifier and oxygen machine overwhelmed my senses.

Propped up on a recliner chair sat John Howard. Mr. Howard and I reviewed his medical condition and proceeded to look at the broken plate. The appliance turned out to be a partial denture with a pair of broken clips. To make matters worse, two large pieces of acrylic were missing. Repair would be impossible.

The equipment I was able to bring that day was inadequate to prepare a new partial denture, so I promised to return the next day. On my way out, Mr. Howard, who hadn't spoken much, reminded me in a rasping voice how long it had been since he had eaten properly.

The following day, after an overwhelming schedule at my private practice, I was again a little late in getting to the Howards. As I hurried from my car to their apartment, I turned a corner and nearly stumbled into the teenagers from the day before.

One stepped forward to accost me but was immediately interrupted. "Back down, man, he's seeing the Colonel," said the biggest.

I continued on my way and arrived to find Annie at the door. Saying hello to John, I started taking impressions and bites. As I cleaned up in Annie's kitchen, she told me of John's service record in the Army; he had been a colonel. "The Colonel" was quite proud of his accomplishments, and many pictures of a much younger man in uniform lined the hallway.

When I got back to my patient, I assured him I'd have his new teeth in less than a week. He reminded me again of his desire to eat steak. On my way out, I felt the urge to give him a salute—it must have been all the military conversation. He acknowledged my gesture with a curt nod.

About a week later, I looked forward to seeing the Howards again. Thinking about the neighborhood where they lived, though, brought on very real apprehension. I had scheduled the final appointment much later in the day than the previous appointments.

It was dark when I arrived, so I hurried to the Howards, glad to know I'd soon be finished with this case. As I rounded the corner, my young friends were waiting, nearly causing me to drop the new teeth. After a nervous moment, one finally said, "Stand clear, he has the Colonel's teeth." By the time I arrived at the Howards, followed closely by the teenagers, my heartbeat had returned to normal.

The Colonel was not in good spirits, Annie explained. It had been a particularly difficult day for his comfort. I couldn't wait to try in the denture. After donning mask and gloves, I assured the Colonel he would soon be enjoying solid food again. Naturally, as I went to try the denture, it wouldn't fit.

The Colonel couldn't hold back his frustration. Since it was summer in New England, the front door was open with only the screen door separating us from the busy courtyard. The Colonel's loudly voiced dissatisfaction carried through the door, and the loitering teens outside asked if everything was alright. Annie reassured them. I suddenly sensed the need to finish this treatment as quickly as possible and get out of there. I realized that the fit of a dental appliance fabricated in a distant lab might determine if I made it back to my car in one piece that night.

After several moments of self-doubt and a few minor adjustments, the partial fit his gums beautifully. The look on the Colonel's face could only be described as a combination of surprise and relief. Enthralled at having the missing teeth replaced, it took some heavy persuasion before he agreed to let me remove the denture one more time for a final bite adjustment.

nce the post-treatment instructions were given, I assured Annie and John Howard that I would be at their disposal in the weeks ahead. After good-byes were exchanged and I was halfway to the door, Mr. Howard called out in the rasp that served as his voice, "Doc!"

I turned to see my patient offering a formal military salute. As he wheezed, "Thank you," I caught the glint of a tear in Colonel Howard's eye. I returned the salute and briskly walked to my car.

It's strange, but on my ride back to the office I couldn't help but hope for another call to the wrong side of town. ❤

—Christopher Freyermuth, DMD

Alice

The most important medicine is tender love and care.

—Mother Teresa

lice, age 73 at the time, was sent to our dental office to have us attempt cleaning her teeth. Her medical doctor was trying to solve her septicemia (blood poisoning) problem and thought that the severe tartar buildup on her teeth might be contributing to this medical situation.

I guided Alice's wheelchair into one of our operatories. The nurse accompanying Alice said, "Good luck. I don't think you will be able to do anything, but her doctor wants you to try."

Seeing that this would be an extremely difficult situation, I went into the other operatory to tell the hygienist she wouldn't be able to handle this one on her own and that it would take both of us. I did not offer further explanation as she was still with another patient.

Going back in with Alice and seeing the blank stare and the constant chewing motion, I wondered about this myself. She did not seem to understand anything that was said to her.

Jayne, the bubbly hygienist at our office, walked into the room (without even looking at Alice) saying "Hi, Alice, how are you doing?" It just struck me funny, and I burst out laughing— I was definitely not laughing at Alice.

When I laughed, a big smile broke out on Alice's beautiful

face and she opened real wide. Every time I laughed, Alice would smile big and open wide, and we could clean some more of her teeth. By the end of this difficult appointment, Jayne and I were both crying because somehow this wonderful lady had touched our hearts.

The following day, we visited the nursing home to check on Alice. When we went into her room and she heard our voices, a large smile appeared on her face. We continued these visits several times a week. She went from flinching when we touched her to leaning toward us, desiring a loving touch. She went from pulling her hair out (she had almost no hair at all on either side of her head when we first met her) to having a full head of hair. She went from the blank stare to being responsive to our voices. She can now even push the buttons on children's songbooks to play music. Even though she may still live in her own little world, I know we are a part of it.

any times, all it takes for a person to feel human is for someone else to love them and show that they care. Besides the lesson of love, another lesson I learned is that many of us may have special gifts inside of us that God would like us to share. Who would have ever thought that all of this could have come from one dental visit? I am very grateful to this remarkable woman. Because of her, I have befriended many residents at the nursing home. I see all of them on a regular basis and believe I have made a difference in their lives. They have definitely touched my heart...especially Alice! ❤

—Marla Leibfried, CDA

On Call for Christmas

*The capacity to care is what gives life
its deepest meaning and significance.*

—Pablo Casals

t was Christmas Eve, and I had drawn the short straw; now I was the "on-call doctor" for our dental group.

"Hey, don't worry," advised my colleague as he handed me the pager. "Everyone is so busy with their own Christmas plans, no one will ever call." I hoped he was right.

As I drove home, my car radio played "I'll be home for Christmas," and I began to sing along: "I'm on call for Christmas, you can count on me."

When I walked through our front door, there was a whirlwind of activity as my wife finished preparations for the special family dinner with our visiting relatives. Finally, we sat down to the first course of baked acorn squash soup. No sooner had the bowls been removed and the main course served than the beep of the pager jolted me.

"Who could be calling on Christmas Eve?" I wondered with more than a little irritation. I quickly cleaned my plate but really didn't taste another bite. Excusing myself, I reluctantly dialed the number on my pager.

Between sobs, the woman who answered the phone said she had started dialing every dentist in the phone book and that I was the only one to call her back. She told me she had broken a tooth a few weeks earlier and was now in excruciating pain.

"It sounds like you probably need a root canal," I explained. "I'll meet you at my office in 45 minutes." Knowing it would ruin Christmas Eve with my family, I kicked myself for agreeing to make such a special accommodation for someone who wasn't even a patient of mine. With 30 minutes to drive to the office, perhaps an hour or more with the patient, and another 30 minutes to drive home, it would be after 10 o'clock before I returned to my family.

"What is it?" asked my wife.

"Some idiot who's had a problem for weeks now and has just decided on Christmas Eve that it needs to be fixed!" I hollered over my shoulder as I stormed out of the house.

On the drive to the office, I heard that song on the car radio again and joined in: "I'm on call for Christmas, you can count on me...." I furiously pounded the steering wheel as I sang.

When I arrived at the office and began to unlock the front door, I heard someone approaching. I turned and saw a *very* pregnant woman walking slowly toward me.

"Are you Mary?" I asked.

"Yes, Doctor, thank you for coming out to help me," she began.

"When are you due?" I inquired.

"Any minute now," she explained.

My anger quickly vanished and I felt ashamed for being so upset by this emergency. "Well, come on in. At least we'll get your tooth fixed up." Her broken tooth was badly decayed and would clearly need root canal treatment. I explained that I would start the procedure that evening and finish after her baby was delivered. And so, Mary, the unborn babe, and I spent Christmas Eve together treating a bad tooth.

As I worked, I thought of another time, another Mary, and the unborn Jesus. They would have had a very bad night that first Christmas Eve had it not been for the kindness of a stranger—a caring innkeeper who took pity on them and let them use his stable.

"Okay, Tylenol should take care of any pain from the procedure. I think you'll do just fine. Give me a call in a few weeks and we'll finish the root canal," I told Mary.

"Thank you very much for helping me," she replied. "I'm sorry I ruined your Christmas."

uined? Well, the evening had not turned out like I expected, but I felt as though I had been called on to play the modern role of the kindly innkeeper— to help Mary in her hour of need. Ruined? No, my Christmas Eve had been *enriched*. In some ways it was almost like being part of the First Christmas. ♥

—Thomas G. Dwyer, DDS, MS

Home for Christmas Dinner

Cinnamon, nutmeg—steaming ginger teas
December is a potpourri, a winter-scented breeze
Cedar branches, fir trees—my memories impart
And take me home—to Christmas!
On the perfume of the heart

—From "Cinnamon Christmas" by S.G. Cooley

t was the Friday before Christmas, and I was trying to complete all my work so that I could leave for the holiday. We had plans, important plans. Christmas dinner: a feast of delights for the eye and the palate. In my heart, I could hear the laughter and see the beloved faces that would soon ring our dining room table: my sisters and brothers and my beautiful mother. This is what I work and live for—the celebration of faith with my family.

I told the dental clinic receptionist I couldn't possibly accommodate one more drop-in. But as I turned to step back into my office, I saw the stoic face of a waiting child. It was José. He was 11, with large brown eyes and a clenched set to his jaw. José was in obvious pain. And I was in a hurry.

I checked the chart and found that José had been referred to our health center by an ER physician. The doctor had prescribed an excellent medication for pediatric pain control, and given enough time to kick in, the medicine should keep the boy comfortable through the weekend. That's what I told the receptionist who, in turn, relayed the message to José and his mother. Moments later, parent and child left the clinic.

And then, while visions of sugarplums danced in my head, I calmly repeated that professional opinion to my conscience.

Five minutes later, I was on the phone. While I dialed José's mother, I remembered another child from long ago, a little girl with a toothache. Curled into a knot of pain, she cried on her mother's couch—my mother's couch—until the pillows were wet with my tears.

When nobody answered, I waited another five minutes— an eternity—before calling again. Mercifully, Mrs. Lopez answered.

I wasted no time with apologies. "Bring your son back to the clinic immediately, and I'll be here to meet you." How could I eat dinner, how could I look into the eyes of my nephews—and not see José?

We took care of that tooth. And José took care of my soul. For what little time I sacrificed, he gave me a beautiful, everlasting Christmas present.

This very young man has become a model patient. I grin ear to ear while he stands in my operatory and lectures his siblings on brushing and flossing. The Lopez family now has its own in-residence, oral hygiene advocate.

José, this story is for you, my friend. And for all our José's, whose precious teeth suffer from simple neglect and finally rebel in pain and infection. José, I am so proud of you. And I thank you for your bright smile and your concern for your brother and sister.

entistry is more than a physical practice. My personal philosophy is influenced by writers and poets who pass on their experience in prose and verse. The late Thomas Merton, a Trappist monk and author with a worldwide following, is a favorite of mine.

Merton's simple axiom was this:

> *The thing to do when you have made a mistake is not to give up what you were doing and start something altogether new, but to start over again with the thing you began badly and try, for the love of God, to do it well.*

Merton's message is the call of my life: to live it well, to do things well. When I succeed in that goal, then I can walk into our dining room, behold the faces I love, and enjoy the pungent sweetness of home. That's when I whisper aloud in my heart, "God bless us—every one." ♥

—Pamela Arbuckle Alston, DDS, FACD

Sarah

pon graduation, most dental hygienists choose the traditional setting of a private dental practice. However, I learned that there are other career options, and my calling was to public health where I have spent my entire career.

Many years ago, I routinely performed dental exams on elementary school students in my health unit district. A portable dental chair and light was carried into each school and assembled in the medical room—or in some cases, the library, the music room, or even the storage room. Along with the equipment, I had enough mirrors and explorers to examine up to 120 children in a single day. My district had 27 schools, and I conducted these exams for many years. Needless to say I saw thousands of children annually, but I especially remember one little girl whom I'll call Sarah.

A kindergarten student, Sarah wore a kerchief on her head in an attempt to hide the signs of hair loss. As she sat down in my chair and leaned back, I noticed that her movements were stiff. Sarah's dress draped her little frame, and I could see the outline of a body cast covering her torso. As I performed the exam, I remarked that she had a "wiggly tooth." I told her that soon it would fall out and be replaced by a permanent tooth. With a mirror, I showed Sarah which tooth was loose; and she gave it a wiggle with her tongue.

Since Sarah was my last student of the day, I walked

back to her classroom with her to give the teacher the referral forms. As we approached the room, the teacher was standing in the doorway. Sarah skipped up to her and shared the wonderful news.

"I have a wiggly tooth, and I didn't even know it!" she exclaimed as she hugged her teacher.

 mall things we take for granted were big events for Sarah. The natural evolution of losing a baby tooth is a wonder lost on many of us, but not for Sarah. Although her body was only performing a natural function, to a child who has suffered through the unnatural consequences of cancer, it was an event to celebrate.

I looked forward to seeing Sarah again the following year when she would have been in grade one. Her spirit was something I wanted to experience again. The following September, when the class lists from the schools arrived, I looked for Sarah's name. I could not find her.

When I went to the school, I did not ask about Sarah. I wanted to be able to believe that she had moved. It was reasonable that her family might move to the city to be closer to Children's Hospital. That was 15 years ago. I still imagine Sarah as alive and well—another child who was able to beat the ravages of cancer. ♥

—Sharon Louise Melanson, RDH

Children of Bosnia

What does Love look like? It has hands to help others.
It has feet to hasten to the poor and needy.
It has eyes to see misery and want.
It has ears to hear the sighs and sorrows of fellow men.
That is what Love looks like.

—Saint Augustine

ric, I have a couple of kids here from Bosnia. They each have severe dental decay and require the removal of a lot of teeth. Can you fit them in next week?" inquired Dr. D.T. Brown.

"No problem D.T.; I'll have Leslie, our patient coordinator, rearrange Tuesday's schedule." Since I'm a specialist in oral and maxillofacial surgery, it is not unusual for me to receive such requests. Little did I know that this particular Tuesday would be different from all the previous Tuesdays I've experienced in 17 years of private practice.

Reflecting on the call I had just received, I thought to myself, "Every town needs a dentist like D.T. Brown, a man with a heart of gold." Whether he's providing hot meals for the homeless or painting parking meters in the downtown area, he's always doing something for somebody. D.T. had explained that these Bosnian children were scheduled to undergo complex orthopedic reconstructive surgery by Dr. Victor Macko in the coming weeks. The boy had sustained a nasty knee injury, and the girl had injured both her foot and leg when a soldier in the Bosnian army threw a grenade into their home. Since the children were Serbian and their parents did not trust the Bosnian dentists, they had developed terrible dental infections due to simple neglect. It was important that the infection in their jaws be corrected before the orthopedic surgery; otherwise, germs in the mouth could easily travel through the blood and infect the surgical sites.

Tuesday morning, my staff and I met Milos Supica. For years, Milos has been responsible for rescuing children from war-torn Bosnia. He arranges transportation, housing, and the provision of surgical care when necessary. He introduced us to Milandinka, age 12, and Mladen, age eight. Each child was given a Beanie Baby that my staff members had purchased specially for them. The children's mother stood silently by their side, her eyes suggesting a mixture of grief and hope. My examination confirmed that many of the children's primary and permanent teeth were badly decayed and beyond repair. Removal was the only possible option. Milos translated, and we decided to treat eight-year-old Mladen first. Milos commented, "The boy will be no problem, but I am worried about the girl."

Clutching his Beanie Baby, Mladen limped into the operating room. The relaxing nitrous oxide "laughing gas" rapidly entered his lungs; a catheter was placed into his right arm; and intravenous anesthesia quickly rendered Mladen unconscious. He welcomed the sleep, and the surgery was soon over.

After placing Mladen on the recovery bed, Tammi and Kandi, my surgical staff, assisted Milandinka to the operatory room. The girl was tearful, and there was rapid conversation with Milos translating as she lay on the operating chair. Milandinka needed to have three permanent molars and seven baby teeth removed. Her eyes darted about, filled with fear as we attempted to introduce the needle into her right arm. She struggled and cried.

Her brother left the recovery bed and tried to comfort his sister, "Look, my teeth are pulled. He won't hurt you, trust him." There was a rapid exchange of words between Milos and Milandinka as we held her in place.

It was then that Milandinka exclaimed, "What did I do to deserve this? Why am I being punished? I should have died with the others!"

After Milos translated, his face was drained and lost all color. All of us were stunned—overwhelmed with grief and sorrow. Fearful that the sensitive Milos might pass out, we escorted him to the recovery room.

Tammi, Kandi, and I wiped tears from our eyes and thought, "How could this beautiful child wish she had died?" Just about then the anesthetics started to take effect, and Milandinka fell silently asleep. Her nightmare was at an end.

After the procedures were completed and Tammi and Kandi walked the children to their car, Milos hugged Tammi and said, "God bless you."

That evening, I called Milos to check on my little patients. They each came to the phone and, in their best English, said, "Thank you, Dr. Wall."

Needless to say, that Tuesday was a very emotional day for all of us; my staff and I will never be the same. That brief insight into the war in Bosnia gave us a great appreciation of our life here in the U.S.A.

n Thanksgiving Day, our local newspaper, *The Record*, ran a front-page story about Milos and the children from Bosnia. Dr. Macko's five-hour operation on Milandinka's foot was a success, and both children were well on their way to recovery! ♥

—Eric B. Wall, DDS; Leslie Cruz;
Tammi Holley; and Kandi Vargas

Steve

*I wanted a perfect ending.... Now I've learned, the hard way,
that some poems don't rhyme, and some stories don't have a
clear beginning, middle, and end. Life is about not knowing,
having to change, taking the moment and making the best of it,
without knowing what's going to happen next.*

—Gilda Radner

 had been practicing at the Phoenix, Arizona, HIV clinic for just a few months when Steve came in for dental hygiene therapy. Just a few minutes in his presence revealed an arrogant young man of about 25 with a huge chip on his shoulder. He took his own sweet time sitting in my chair and, when he finally did, announced with a condescending air that I had only 30 minutes to "clean his teeth."

My first reaction was, "Why did he have to come in on my day?" I've always had a problem with patients who acted as if they were doing me a favor by showing up. It wasn't that I didn't like practicing at the clinic—I thoroughly enjoyed working there. It was 1994 and the HIV epidemic was still going strong. I had practiced dental hygiene in a variety of locations for 20 years, and this clinic was proving to be my favorite. The patients were down-to-earth, friendly, and appreciative. I'd become good friends with many of them. Most of my patients were plagued with opportunistic infections and diseases, but their spirits were strong and their attitudes were positive.

Every one of the patients I treated was confident that he would be the one who beat the odds to overcome this terrible disease. And I hoped that each of them would be the person that did it. They all treated me with respect and courtesy, and I, in turn, respected each of them for their vitality and their kindness.

It appeared to me that Steve, however, was not going to be one of the individuals that I particularly liked. I took his blood pressure and reviewed his medical history. Steve's health was declining rapidly. He had numerous opportunistic infections and other indications that he was not going to live much longer, despite his healthy appearance. When I completed his oral exam it was clear that 30 minutes would not be enough for any meaningful treatment.

"Steve, it looks as if I will probably need numerous appointments to complete your treatment." I explained to him why the extra time was necessary, describing his oral condition and all the calculus that was present, as well as the severe inflammation present throughout his gums. He not only needed treatment, he also needed instruction on oral hygiene procedures that would make his mouth healthy and comfortable again.

"No. You had 30 minutes today, and you've already wasted half of that. Get it done today. I'm not coming back."

I wasn't looking for an argument, so I started my treatment, having only 15 minutes left of his "30-minute appointment." I touched his teeth gently with my instruments and very slowly and gingerly allowed my probe to go under his gumline. Steve didn't like that and made a move to push my hands away.

"That hurts badly. I'm leaving."

With that statement, I decided it was probably best to forget dental hygiene treatment and just talk to Steve. The HIV clinic was a free service, and I was fortunate that I could opt for no treatment right then. I got a mirror and showed him everything in his mouth. I explained to him why his gums were bleeding and why they hurt. I told him that I wouldn't begin any treatment unless he wanted me to. And quite honestly, had he agreed to continue, I would have scheduled him for one of the days that I wouldn't be there. His entire attitude bothered me—he was rude, condescending, and thoroughly unpleasant.

Steve continued to be smug but, when he got up to leave, he shook my hand. I softened a little and asked him to come back in a few weeks if he wanted me to work on him. I was pretty certain, though, that I wouldn't see him in the clinic again.

Surprisingly, he was back within a week, still with a chip on his shoulder and looking less healthy. But this time he'd scheduled a 90-minute appointment. He was a bit irritated when I told him that we would need several more 90-minute sessions to complete the job, but he reluctantly agreed. He did his best to give me a hard time all the while I worked on him, but by this time I knew he was bluffing. "All bark and no bite," I figured. He was becoming almost likeable.

Steve didn't make his next appointment and I assumed he was just going to forget about coming back. Later that day I learned that on his way to the clinic, he'd collapsed and been rushed to the hospital. Pneumonia.

It was two months before Steve came to the clinic again. He looked gaunt, he looked tired, and he'd lost the spark in his eye that was so much a part of both his anger and his charm. But he was determined to continue his treatment. This time he was a model patient, though he only had the strength to sit in my chair for 30 minutes. We decided he could come in whenever he was able, and I would work on him as long as he was comfortable.

Over the next three months, I got to know Steve well. He was adamant about coming in for all his appointments, but he was going downhill fast. Our relationship evolved from tolerance for one another to friendship. He told me about his family, particularly his mother who was taking care of him. He felt he was a burden to her, but I could tell by the way he talked that they were very close and that she was taking good care of her precious and much-loved son.

Finally, we got to the point where Steve needed only one more appointment. That day I went into the clinic's reception area to get him. He was in a wheelchair this time with his mother sitting next to him holding his hand. A thin man to begin with, he had lost more than 30 pounds since I started treating him and looked ashen. But Steve had on the loudest pair of pants I had ever seen—red with intensely bright colors splashed all over. He smiled at me weakly but beamed when I told him I thought he looked great in those pants. His mother flashed me a look of gratitude, tears moistening her eyes.

This time Steve could barely stay upright in my chair. He was very sick and in a great deal of pain. But he told me that he wouldn't leave until I'd completed that day's treatment. He wanted to know that each and every tooth in his mouth was as clean and healthy as it could be.

Although it wasn't the truth, after a few minutes' work I told him we were done. His mother touched my arm, and I knew I'd lifted a huge burden from her shoulders—and from Steve's.

teve died three weeks later. It took some time for me to realize this, but I now know that his early defiance arose from a need to say, "This is still my life. I am still in control." As his illness progressed and his strength ebbed, I believe Steve's priorities changed. I think that the simple act of making it through treatment became one of his final goals and accomplishments. But it wasn't his only accomplishment. I look at my challenging patients a little differently now. And I remember Steve. ♥

—Debby Kurtz-Weidinger, RDH, MEd

Seek and Ye Shall Find

I can't explain it. All I know is that prayer works.

—Norman Cousins

he voice on the phone sounded urgent. It was after 10:00 PM, and Susan was calling our home from the emergency room. Her husband, Brian, had taken a bicycle ride about three hours earlier and had slid on fine pea-gravel while turning a corner. Not only did he have multiple scrapes, bruises, and lacerations over various parts of his body, he had also broken several teeth and was missing one front tooth altogether!

Susan's request was to see if I would go to the site of the accident and look for the missing tooth in the hope of re-implanting it.

Several hours had already passed, and I knew that the odds of finding the tooth—much less saving it—were quite slim. Hoping to determine the exact location of the accident, I called the police station, but was told that the officer who had been at the scene was off duty.

With only an address near the accident site, a prayer, and a flashlight, I started my search. In the shadowy darkness, randomly pierced by the headlights of passing cars, the pea-sized gravel on the roadside looked much the same color and size as a human tooth.

More than an hour later, just as I was ready to give up,

the first miracle happened—my flashlight shone on the tooth! I picked it up, drove to my office, performed a root canal on the tooth, and placed it in a saline solution. At the hospital, I offered another prayer and re-implanted the tooth into Brian's mouth.

It's now been ten years, and a second miracle has manifested itself—Brian still has his original tooth! ❤

—Richard L. Parker, DDS

4

A FULFILLING CAREER

Open your eyes and look for some man,
or some work for the sake of men
which needs a little time,
a little sympathy, a little sociability.
It is needed in every nook and corner.
Therefore, search for some place
where you may invest your humanity.

—Albert Schweitzer

Sweet Sixteen

All the great things are simple,
and many can be expressed in a single word:
freedom, justice, honor, duty, mercy, faith, hope, love.

—Winston Churchill

elicity Jacobs rarely smiled. If she did, a practiced hand would fly to her face, covering the gaps between her front teeth. Felicity was a model patient, an expert with toothbrush and floss. But the measured spaces between her teeth gave her smile all the grace of a picket fence.

When the sight of your own smile breaks your heart, your world is not a very bright place. Especially, if you're 15. As I prepared to solve Felicity's dilemma, I remembered where I was at her age.

On the morning of my sixteenth birthday, my parents took us all to a train station—an *East German* train station. I was a child of the Cold War and grew up behind the line in Europe that Winston Churchill called an Iron Curtain.

Behind that curtain you would have found the Neumarker family, my parents, my brother, Rainer, and me. The Communist regime was a brooding threat to everyone. Like all good mothers and fathers, my parents wanted their children to be healthy, happy—and *free*. It was much later in my life before I knew that the events of my sixteenth birthday had been three years in the planning.

There was no party. But there was a cover story, a smoke screen to throw off the neighborhood spies. And there was an escape attempt—to cast off the manacles of Communism.

Mother and Father had bundled us all together for what the neighbors were told was *"a holiday on the Baltic Sea."* Before dawn, we made our way to the station.

When you traveled in the old Soviet satellite nations, there were guards carrying submachine guns, police examining travel documents, on-the-spot interrogations—you walked every day through a minefield of martial law. The first part of our trip was halted at a checkpoint just outside East Berlin while papers were examined and each adult was questioned.

Among those most closely interrogated was my father. Father was escorted off the train and taken to the side of the tracks. In deathly silence, beside the ready barrels of two submachine guns, my father faced Russian and East German guards.

"Herr Neumarker, just how is it that a machinist like yourself can afford such travel?"

My face pressed against the window glass, I watched as Father gave the performance of his life.

"My sons are good children...it is not easy, but they deserve a little holiday."

Father knew, and I knew—one slip of the tongue, one misstep, and both my parents would disappear. And the Neumarker children could wake up the next morning in a work camp.

"You don't appear to me to be a happy traveler, Herr Neumarker. Something tells me your boys will never see the Baltic."

I held my breath while my father flawlessly pleaded the innocence of our "vacation."

Father was released. The waiting train resumed its journey, taking us into the heart of East Berlin.

It was supposed to be a three-hour layover. But my parents had other plans.

The guard was right: we never saw the Baltic.

Mother took Rainer and slipped down to the subway that was the conduit between Communist East Berlin and West Berlin, political gateway to the free republic of West Germany.

At the checkpoint, Mother told a partial truth: she was only escorting her son for a brief, legal visit with relatives. The guards let them go. Once across, Mother took Rainer to a West Berlin safe house where they anxiously waited for me and Father.

When Father believed Mother and Rainer were safe in the western sector, he picked up the solitary suitcase containing all our worldly possessions, took my hand, and together we, too, crossed the border into a new life. We were free.

"Happy Birthday, Rudi!"

y American sons ask me to repeat this story for them every now and then. The last time they heard it was this evening when I told them about Felicity, the girl with the hiding face. I spent two hours with my young patient, erasing all the gaps between her teeth with composite fillings. When a dazzling smile greeted her in the mirror, she cried. Her mother cried, my assistant cried! I have to admit the whole thing choked me up, too. We adults were privileged to be present as a child's world became a brighter place. My work was a gift from her mother: it was Felicity's sixteenth birthday.

On the day I turned 16, my world became a brighter place. I could only dream of immigrating to America, learning a new language, graduating from high school, and earning a doctorate in dentistry. Freedom is a wonderful thing.

In freedom, we can make our dreams come true. My profession permits me to cure disease and teach good dental hygiene. Dentists have so many opportunities to minister to patients' practical needs, revealing the secrets of sweet breath and bright smiles. Every single day, I am humbled with gratitude for the opportunity to serve my patients. And every

evening I thank God for the deep satisfaction that I draw from
this work.

n bedtime prayers, I always remember my patients.
Tonight, I'll think of one in particular who lit up my
office with the brilliance of her smile: *Felicity,
thank you for your contribution to my life. I dedicate
this story to you. There's just one thing I have to add...
Happy Birthday, my young friend! Isn't 16 sweet?* ♥

—Rudi Neumarker, DDS
As told to Don Dible

Giving and Receiving

Don't expect the best gifts to come wrapped in pretty paper.
—H. Jackson Brown

fter graduating from the University of Detroit's dental hygiene program, I divided my practice between a community dental clinic and a rehabilitation institute, both in rural western Michigan. School had pumped me full of high ideals, but working in the real world soon deflated my noble notions. I started out with plans to clean up the mouths of everyone in my little corner of the world but soon discovered that the process relies heavily on cooperation from patients. Sadly, most of the patients I saw didn't share my enthusiasm.

Three dental hygienists worked with three dentists at the clinic providing much needed care to the indigent residents in three neighboring counties. Some of the families living along the back roads were as poor as dirt—and wore it on their clothes and faces. One day after lunch, we awaited the arrival of a Medicaid family of six brothers; each hygienist was scheduled to treat two boys. Imagine six blond heads with greasy, stringy hair; sweet looking, dirt-streaked faces; and filthy, ripped clothing. One boy had no shoes, and his feet were as black as coal dust. Their oral hygiene rivaled their personal hygiene.

The oldest of the six, Norman, was a sullen young man of about 13. In striking up a conversation, the boy told me his family shared one toothbrush among all eight members and that it had been a gift to one of the brothers by a hygienist at school during Children's Dental Health Month. My heart went out to this poor family. Their struggle in life seemed more difficult than I could ever imagine. I wondered what it must be like to be so hungry you eat the stale bread sent over by neighbors for your small flock of ducks.

I gave Norman and one of his brothers my best care, spending a great deal of time on oral hygiene instructions. Each received a new toothbrush with my ultimatum not to let anyone else use it—the brushes were for their personal, exclusive, individual use. I told the boys those brushes were my gifts to them and that their gifts back to me would be to use the brushes regularly and to take good care of their teeth. At the end of this particular day, I remember feeling the frustration of knowing that, once again, my efforts at helping had fallen on deaf ears.

About two weeks later, I was driving home as usual after a day of work at the rehabilitation institute. Due to a construction project, I had to take a short detour down one back road and return to the main highway on another. On the last leg of the detour, I noticed an old yellow school bus resting on cinder blocks in a clearing about 100 feet off the road. Someone had hung red gingham curtains in the windows giving the bus a lived-in appearance.

A closer look revealed that a family had made it their home. Just the thought of someone living in a school bus without running water, heat, or electricity—especially in Michigan during the harsh winters—was enough to make my toes freeze right off. Two disheveled, blond-headed boys were roughhousing in front of the bus and I recognized one as Norman, my patient from the clinic.

I pulled onto the shoulder and backed up in front of the makeshift house. It took a few minutes before I got his attention; then I yelled, "Hey, Norman! Have you been brushing your teeth? I'm counting on you to take care of your teeth and to help your little brothers take care of theirs too."

Norman was obviously stunned by my sudden appearance and it took several seconds for him to answer. We exchanged a few pleasantries; and then I resumed my journey home, laughing about his reaction to my impromptu house call.

Over time, I forgot about Norman and his brothers and continued to grow more disillusioned with my work. I had always thought that as a dental hygienist I would touch lives and improve my patients' overall wellbeing, but time proved how naïve that expectation was. My patients just seemed bored and uninterested, showing up every six months with their mouths in just as bad shape as—if not worse than—on the previous visit. I began to seriously consider a different line of work, one that could provide me with a greater sense of personal fulfillment.

bout two months into my new job search, Norman and his brothers returned to the clinic for their recall appointments. I made sure that Norman was on my schedule so that I could chart his oral hygiene progress. After a quick examination, I could tell he had done a bang-up job of brushing his teeth. I said, "Why, Norman, just look at this! Your teeth and gums are in great shape! I'm so proud of you. You were actually listening to me."

In response, this normally silent young man said, "I was hoping you'd notice. I did it for you. It's my gift, remember?"

Well Norman, my boy, you gave me one incredible gift. On that day, I learned the best gifts are not bought with money. Finally, I had touched someone's life and—surprise of all surprises—he had touched mine. Innocent words, spoken in truth, had a profound effect on me because here I am, 24 years later, hanging on to the memory of that gift and providing oral hygiene instructions to all who will listen. ♥

—Becky Sroda, RDH, MS

You *Do* Make a Difference!

If someone listens, or stretches out a hand, or whispers a
kind word of encouragement, or attempts to understand
a lonely person, extraordinary things begin to happen.

—Loretta Girzatlis

ave you ever thought that you are unable to change things—that nothing you do could *possibly* make a difference in the life of another person? I want to tell you about Margaret, a Canadian woman who made a difference. She changed *forever* the life of a teenager.

I remember that impatient girl. Although "Danni" was loved and cherished by her mom and dad, she left home at 16 to seek her own way. Raised in a family where both young parents wore dentures, she had never been to a dental office. But soon after asserting her independence, Danni faced the looming challenge of going to the dentist...alone.

As she timidly entered the reception area, the girl's fear spilled over into quiet tears. And then a soft voice called her name. *"Danni—I'm ready for you."* It was Margaret.

In this innovative private practice in Winnipeg, Margaret was a dental assistant assigned to instruct new patients in a preventive dental-care program. Danni's years without regular visits to the dentist had left scars throughout her mouth. The plaque prevention regimen she entered was designed to build a new patient ethic of conscientious homecare. For Danni, it proved to be an overwhelming success.

As the program was structured, Danni didn't see the dentist at the first appointment...or even the next. In fact, for two solid weeks Danni visited the office every day and, in 15-minute sessions with Margaret, mastered the simple arts of brushing and flossing. Soon there was a dramatic change in her gums—they no longer bled every time she brushed. For the first time since leaving home, Danni felt secure and confident.

Following Margaret's orientation cycle, the dentist began clinical restoration of the teenager's eager smile. Visits were frequent, but as long as faithful Margaret was on hand to explain everything as it was happening, Danni was able to relax. And her dental health improved by measurable increments.

Progressive treatment affords patients and practitioners a precious bonus: the opportunity to share more than dental history. Danni began to talk about going back to school. She knew she wanted a job that would include working with people, but she couldn't decide what she was interested in.

"Why not take dental assisting?" Margaret offered.

Danni listened—*and she acted.*

t's been more than 20 years since that once-frightened girl graduated as a registered dental assistant. Subsequently, she worked in general and specialty practices before becoming an educational technologist in a dental assisting program in Calgary.

As Danni's life moved onward—and westward—she lost contact with her mentor. But I can assure you of this: Margaret was one person who made a significant difference in a young life. I know she did...*I* am "Danni." ❤

—Danelle Fulawka, RDA
2001 President
Canadian Dental Assistants' Association

A Mother's Faith

The dedicated life is the life worth living.

—Annie Dillard

emember getting your driver's license? Remember what a feeling of grown-up freedom you felt? My 16-year-old son just left alone with the car for the first time. He is so full of excitement; I am so full of terror. He is a wonderful, responsible young man who appreciates all he is and all he has. He knows that our lives could have been much different than they are now.

Today, I'm a 39-year-old hygienist who's worked in the dental field for 23 years. One morning some years ago, I awoke terrified, faced with the realization that I was a newly divorced parent with two small children. My daughter was ill with asthma, and my dad was dying of emphysema. With frequent hospital visits for my daughter, the loss of medical insurance, and no child support, I was told, gently yet firmly, that I would have to go on public assistance so that the children could have medical coverage.

I cannot express in words my deep shame and sadness at where I was in my life and the concern I felt about what would become of my beautiful, innocent children and me. I thank God for my children; they kept me on a straight path. I also thank my friends, especially Candee and her family, who stayed by my side, and my dearest friend, Michael, who gave

me the strength to deal with all the other little problems that
kept creeping into my life.

 had many ideas as to what I could do to support
my children, but there was only one thing I really
wanted to do—go back to school and study dental
hygiene. It was something I had always dreamed of
but never thought I could accomplish. After much pondering,
I took a deep breath and went to our local community college
to find out what the program would entail. I spoke with the
head of the dental hygiene department who told me there was
no way I would be able to deal with being a single mom, cope
with a sick daughter and a dying father, and expect to complete the required courses. I'm not sure which of my feelings
was stronger, devastation or anger.

My next stop was the administration office where I spoke to
the counselor for a special program to help single moms who
had been out of school for a long time. There I met a woman
named Mara who helped change my life. She said she was a
single mom just like me, but that she had *four* children. She had
received her master's degree and was working on her doctorate,
all while "being there" for her children. She told me I should
never give up because of someone else's innocent ignorance.
She explained that I would have to enroll in a one-year health
certificate program to get back into the swing of education.

After filling out numerous financial aid forms, I enrolled in
college. Full of fear, I desperately hung on to what little self-
esteem I had left. I made a pact with God that I would succeed
for my children—I *would* succeed.

My mom watched the children after school; and my friend,
Jane, her husband, and their children embraced my children as
their own. I don't know what I would have done without their
support. During the first year, my dad passed away. I always
felt so badly that he had to die worrying about me.

A year later, I completed the health certificate program
with a 4.0 grade point average and received an award for out-

standing achievement. I was ready to take on the dental hygiene program; but Mara sat me down and said she wanted me to spend one more year of preparation to get my major science courses taken care of.

I cried all the way home, knowing in my heart that she was right. But I also knew this meant another year on welfare. The stares at the supermarket were really getting to me when I paid for groceries with food stamps. The way I was treated at the hospital when I'd bring my daughter in and present my Medicaid card was also very painful.

I remember my own attitude, many years earlier, when I'd see a person on welfare and think to myself, "They look fine, why should they be on welfare?" I felt so ashamed of the person I used to be all those years ago when I thought my life was perfect and that welfare would never be something I'd have to deal with.

My friend Michael and I dated off and on. His belief in my ability truly encouraged me to forge ahead many times when I didn't think I could study another paper. He knew I couldn't do anything else in my life until I was a self-supporting mom who could make it on her own.

fter my second year of preparation, I was accepted into the dental hygiene program. Every morning, I'd start studying at four so that school wouldn't take time away from my kids. Two years later, I graduated with a 3.9 grade point average and received highest honors. I was inducted into the Phi Theta Kappa National Honor Society; was listed in *Who's Who in American Junior Colleges*; and received the Dental Hygiene Department Award, the Clinical Excellence Award, and the Outstanding Service Award because I had been president of the junior and senior dental hygiene classes.

After passing my national and clinical boards and receiving my license to practice, I ran to the welfare office to say thank you and goodbye. My social workers congratulated me and wished me well.

As I write this story, the local paper is in front of me. My 14-year-old daughter's and 16-year-old son's names are featured in the family section for being on the honor roll at school. I guess all my years of studying had a positive influence on them. They are two of the most wonderful children any parents could ever pray for. I say "parents" because Michael and I are now married and he has adopted my two children.

These days, my work is filled with medical histories, probing, scaling, polishing, flossing, giving homecare instructions, and, most important, listening. Patients are not just teeth and tissue; they are people with fears, concerns, and needs. We never know where they're coming from or where they are going when they leave the office. I always try to hear what they don't say and observe what they do say while being thorough yet gentle. I never leave the office without feeling a sense of fulfillment, satisfaction, and gratitude for the privilege of being able to serve others.

s I finish this story, I can hear my son pulling into the driveway, home safe and sound after his first solo outing with the car. Like any loving parent with two teenagers, I worry endlessly. Next, our wonderful daughter will be venturing into the world. I know she will make it a better place in which to live. Whenever I start to worry about the future, I just remind myself that, with faith, anything is possible. ♥

—Janice M. Dionis, RDH

The Baby Business

*Handle them carefully, for words
have more power than atomic bombs.*

—Pearl Strachan

he relationship between dentist and patient has always been a well-recognized concept; however I never realized just how much until a personal trauma occurred.

To begin, I should explain that I am a pediatric dentist. I chose to pursue this specialty because I've always enjoyed the company of children. They possess true innocence, honesty, originality, and, very often, humor. After my residency program, I was lucky to obtain a job with the Infant Welfare Society of Chicago, a nonprofit organization that provides medical and dental services for the indigent women and children in the city. I love what I do: I utilize my expertise to help those who have nowhere else to go for much-needed services. The dental clinic is well managed and efficient; we accommodate more than 1,300 visits each month for a client base of more than 8,000 patients.

After being hired by the clinic, I got married. Like most newlyweds, I wanted children. Unfortunately, two years elapsed without so much as fertilization. Then one day, during a routine visit to my gynecologist, I was told that an abnormality was found and a biopsy was necessary.

My gynecologist has a rough bedside manner; he is blunt and straight to the point, unlike pediatric dentists. Three days after the biopsy, he called me at the clinic. I was in the middle of a filling on a three-year-old, but I wanted to hear the results of my test. When I got to the phone, he said, "Yeah, I knew it. It's malignant!" At that moment, I was speechless. Then he blurted, "Hey, did you hear me? You have *cancer!*"

Then a number of thoughts filled my head. I wondered, *"How bad is it?" "Can it be removed?" "Will I live?"* But I was so confused that I asked, instead, "What does this mean?"

He then blared, "This means *you're out of the baby business!* Well, I have to go. I'll call you tomorrow with the name of an oncologist," and he hung up before I could say anything else.

As I put the phone down, I was numb. He never answered any of the questions I wanted to ask. Having babies was the furthest thought from my mind; yet he mentioned that. I returned to my patient and completed his filling—tears pooling in my eyes. I began to think, *"Who will complete this patient's much-needed dental work?" "Who will help provide treatment to the large volume of patients we see each day?"*

A week following the biopsy, I was scheduled for immediate surgery to remove the tumor. Radiation therapy was a possible next step. As expected, the surgery made me sterile. The words "you're out of the baby business" kept ringing in my ears. I felt a wave of depression every time I looked down at the large vertical scar that spanned my entire torso. But during my recovery something wonderful happened. I began to receive cards and letters from my patients wishing me to get well and hurry back to work. To this day, I constantly receive words of concern for my health and encouragement about how much my contribution to the clinic means to the families.

 now realize that I will never be without children. I have watched my patients grow up and have children of their own. Those words, *"you're out of the baby business,"* no longer haunt me. Ironically,

I was blessed with the ability to become a pediatric dentist. I have more than 8,000 patients. I am *definitely* "in the baby business!" I am also pleased to say that I have now been cancer-free for more than five years. Even my oncologist thinks this is a miracle...but could it be because of the love and support of *All My Children?* ♥

—Sheila Hall, DDS

A Dedicated
Dental Assistant

The Assistant plans a day ahead
Preparing for the treatment need
Then patiently waits for the go ahead
To follow the dentist's lead.

From the first impression at the door
The patient calls them friend,
To the alginate that begins the plan
To efficiently help them mend.

A smile that keeps the room relaxed,
A word is kindly said.
As the chair leans back and the dental light
Is adjusted overhead.

The Assistant is the core that
Amalgamates the show.
From greet and seat to mix and fix,
This person keeps the flow.

Things quickly put to sterilize.
The sales rep is on the phone.
We hold our own so diligently with
Nerves as plaster stone.

Friend, counselor, repairman, cleaner,
And numerous things untold;
A dedicated Dental Assistant is
More precious than porcelain fused to gold. ♥

—Bess Reeverts CDA, RDA

Friendship

Giving is so often thought of in terms of the gifts we give,
but our greatest giving is of our time, and kindness,
and even comfort for those who need it.
We look on these little things as unimportant—
until we need them.

—Joyce Hilfer

e met in 1965, Ellen and I—two students ready to learn the task and dedication of this profession called dental hygiene. Our friendship became cemented in those challenging two years of education. We developed trust in each other and the ability to share our most intimate thoughts—knowing they would not be repeated. Little did either of us suspect that, later on, it would be our ability to honor a confidence that would allow patients to trust us implicitly.

Life moves along, and in those times there were marriages, children, divorces, deaths, joys, and sorrows; certainly not what either of us had expected. Our friendship remained true and intact—with the ever-growing knowledge that there was more to life than just dental disease. We each performed our "teeth cleaning" tasks and continued to learn while earning the trust of those patients we treated and loved. Through it all, the listening and caring I received from Ellen made a major difference in my life.

One day the call came. "I have to leave; I can do no more.... Please come!" The news was bad—two months to live. My friend's long, quiescent cancer had ravaged in silence. We sat and made a very short list of things to do beginning with a bike ride over the San Francisco Golden Gate Bridge. Just two weeks later, we made the trip.

Ellen's second and last request was to spend time with me, her family, and those she loved. Knowing her son and daughter were to graduate in two years, she made a pact with the Grim Reaper. He gave her a temporary reprieve. After their graduation, Ellen knew the end was drawing near and joined her own family in Idaho.

In the final days, I drove to Boise to be with my friend. When I arrived, she was in bed, frail and pale. As soon as we saw each other, it was decided we had to go out for coffee. With her usual determination, she insisted I help her into the wheelchair. Soon, our small procession headed down the street.

When we returned, Ellen was spent, having made a great last effort to honor our long friendship. I brushed and cleaned her teeth—no self-respecting dental hygienist goes to Heaven without sparkling teeth! I handed her a mirror. She smiled approval and said, "I love you."

My friend Ellen passed on quietly that evening in the arms of her son, surrounded by a small group of those who shared in her love. Her life was a fire whose glow infused all for whom she cared through 30 years of dental hygiene. ❤

—Sandra C. Nelson, RDH, BS, LAP

Northwest Flight 255

orthwest Flight 255 bound for Phoenix, Arizona, crashed just after takeoff from Detroit Metropolitan Airport. The plane slammed onto the I-94 freeway and burst into flames. Rescue workers are searching for survivors."

For me, there was nothing unusual about Sunday, August 16, 1987—until that news bulletin was broadcast. Before then, my interest in forensic dentistry had been merely academic. It just seemed like it might be interesting someday to work with a police agency, or some such group, and put my training and experience to use outside normal dental practice. Now, all of a sudden, the moment had arrived; and I asked myself, *"Do I really want to get involved?"*

I thought long and hard as the media delivered more and more information about the crash. There was only one survivor. A four-year-old girl was miraculously found alive. The other 154 passengers and crew, along with two people on the ground, had perished. The next morning, in a televised news broadcast, authorities discussed the daunting task of identifying the victims.

By Monday evening I had made my decision. I contacted Dr. Allan Warnick, head of the Michigan Dental Association's Forensic Identification Team. "Yes," he said, "we need all the help we can get," and asked me to come down the next morning to the hangar being used as a temporary morgue.

On Tuesday, as I checked in with the security guard and parked my car, I had no idea what to expect or how I would react to these extraordinary circumstances. When I entered the hangar, I was assigned to the postmortem team, handed a mask and latex gloves ("be sure to *double* glove"), and given my instructions. While the gloves offered protection from infection, the mask did nothing to minimize the awful odor.

Hour after hour, for two days, I took turns with my partners—either calling off information from jaws or jaw fragments (fillings, bridge work, missing teeth, etc.) or charting the information called off by my partner. For accuracy, we would then switch places and repeat the process for each specimen. Lunch breaks provided welcome, and much needed, relief. The food was less important than the opportunity to step out into fresh air and walk to the Red Cross tent across the field from the hangar.

Many of the rescue workers and the identification team members suffered psychological problems in varying degrees as a result of their work with the victims of Flight 255. I was fortunate in coming through the ordeal in what I felt was pretty good shape—though I wondered at times why the experience didn't affect me more. I concluded it was partly a matter of mindset. To cope, I imagined I was in an anatomy lab dealing with *specimens*, not parts of human beings.

But my success at emotionally distancing myself from the trauma faltered when I got home in the evenings and read biographical sketches of the victims in the newspaper. I wondered if the jaw I had held in my hand earlier in the day might have belonged to the pretty young girl in the picture on page seven. In short order my instincts asserted themselves again; I stopped reading the paper.

As I thought more about the situation, I decided that the

antemortem team had a much more difficult role in the process. They had to take our charts and make the actual identifications, confronting each family with the grim reality.

Oddly, the most troubling time for me came on my last afternoon when we were asked to walk the crash site. I can't adequately describe the feeling of walking down the eerily deserted Interstate, past torn and blackened plane parts—from small pieces of scrap metal to huge chunks of fuselage. Then there were the little yellow flags scattered all over the site, where bodies and body fragments had been found. Our job, prior to the start of cleanup operations, was to make one final search for body parts that might have been overlooked. I couldn't help noticing the scattered remnants of luggage—clothing that someone would never wear again, a toy that some child would never play with again. A diaper bag for a baby who was gone forever. I was relieved when it was time to return to the hangar.

'm proud of the fact that I was one of the 75 people involved in the identification effort. It took six days, but in the end, every one of the more than 150 victims were identified—the vast majority through dental records. As this is written, 14 years later, I don't think about the crash as often as I once did. However, two aspects of my life have changed forever.

I've become a very attentive airline passenger—I always select a window seat where I can see the wing flaps. Before takeoff, I always pay close attention since pilot error in not setting the wing flaps apparently caused the crash of Flight 255.

The other change is much more subtle—it haunts the shadows of my mind. On those rare occasions when I see little yellow flags on someone's lawn marking the path of under-ground utility lines, my mind jumps back to the crash site and the hangar morgue. I picture myself working on the

If you're enjoying *Love Is the Best Medicine™ for Dental Patients and The Dental Team*, you'll certainly want a copy of

Chicken Soup for the Dental Soul

Sixty-one humorous and inspiring stories for patients, dentists, hygienists, and the entire dental team.

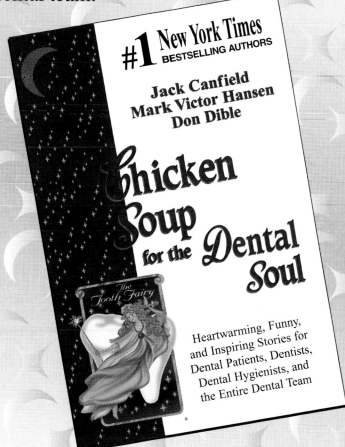

#1 **New York Times** BESTSELLING AUTHORS

Jack Canfield
Mark Victor Hansen
Don Dible

Chicken Soup for the Dental Soul

The Tooth Fairy

Heartwarming, Funny, and Inspiring Stories for Dental Patients, Dentists, Dental Hygienists, and the Entire Dental Team

Although *Chicken Soup for the Dental Soul* is not sold in stores or on the Internet, you may get a single copy or a case by contacting your Patterson Representative or calling:

1-800-637-1140 (in U.S. only).

Love Is the Best Medicine™
for Dental Patients and The Dental Team

The ideal book for your waiting area reading material or as a patient, staff, or fellow professional gift.

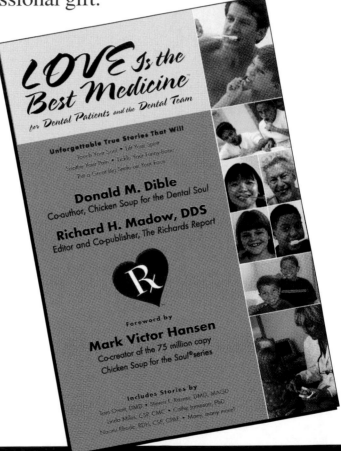

remains of a young child—a three-year-old. That image, still vivid, will never leave me. Nor will I ever forget the contribution modern dentistry has made in identifying lost loved ones, bringing some small comfort to each grieving survivor.

"Would I do it again?" you may ask.

In a heartbeat. ❤

—Robert E. Lavine, DDS

Editor's Note

This story was first submitted by Dr. Lavine in May 2001. As we make the final review of press proofs in late September, less than two weeks have elapsed since the tragic Attack on America in New York; Virginia/Washington, DC; and Pennsylvania. Dr. Lavine has now requested that we add the tribute appearing on the next page—the final change before this book is printed. We consider it a privilege to honor his request.

America's Dental Heroes

I had hoped I would never see another tragedy like Northwest Flight 255—but that now pales in comparison....

There is no shortage of heroes to be found after the terrorist attacks of September 11, 2001 in New York on the World Trade Center, in Washington, DC on the Pentagon, and in Pennsylvania. Among their number are hundreds of dentists (supported by numerous hygienists and dental assistants) from all over the country involved with the mind boggling task of identifying the victims. Their leadership includes Dr. Jeffrey Burkes, Chief Forensic Dentist for the Medical Examiners Office of New York City; Dr. William Yeomans, Director of the Pennsylvania Dental Association's Forensic Dental Identification Team; and Dr. Charles Pemble who heads the Forensic Odontology Team working to identify the victims from the Pentagon.

Many volunteers are working under the auspices of their state dental associations while others, including my Team Leader, Dr. Allan Warnick and Section Leader, Dr. Gary Berman, have been deployed by DMORT (Disaster Mortuary Operational Response Teams). Although they have been asked to work four hour shifts, they are actually putting in back-to-back twelve to fourteen hour days.

While the physical work is difficult, the mental aspect really takes its toll. Dr. Burkes recently ordered the entire Forensic Team to attend a mandatory Psychological Support Session. And yet, hundreds of dentists have already lined up to relieve the current group when their "tour of duty" ends. While they cannot bring the victims back, they can help provide a sense of closure and comfort to the victims' families and friends. The work will go on until it is completed. The goal is still 100% identification. It may take several months. God speed their work.

—R.E.L.

5

MISSION: POSSIBLE

*I expect to pass
through this world but once.
Therefore, if there be any good
that I can do or any kindness
that I can show
to any fellow creature,
let me do it now,
for I shall not pass this way again.*

—William Penn

The Power of Faith

Anger is quieted by a gentle word,
just as fire is quenched by water.

—Megiddo Message

n Haiti, 80% of the population survives in abject poverty, unemployment averages 70%, literacy over the age of 15 is only 45%, and life expectancy at birth is less than 50 years. It is one of the least developed countries in the Western Hemisphere. When I volunteered for a church-sponsored dental mission to this Third World Caribbean nation, I had no idea what I was getting myself into.

Shortly before embarking on my first trip—along with Josh, my 14-year-old son, and Carol, one of my regular staff members—I received a phone call from another dentist. This man had returned to the U.S. several weeks earlier after completing his first mission to Haiti.

He explained that the first patient he had treated in that country was a young woman named Dee Adone. At the time of this initial encounter, he had not yet adjusted to the poverty he later found everywhere in that part of the world, so his vulnerability to Dee's suffering was extreme. In a manner of speaking, he "adopted" this woman for whom he felt only great pity and compassion. He said that Dee was a severe diabetic whose mouth was ravaged with decay and whose abscessed teeth were poisoning her entire body.

While this dentist had properly decided that all of Dee's teeth needed to be extracted, he told me he had removed only half of them during his stay due to her poor health. He concluded his call by asking me to complete the job and remove his patient's remaining teeth.

After I agreed to this follow up treatment, he told me he intended to return to Haiti the next year and make Dee a full set of dentures—no small feat in a country with no dental laboratories!

A month later, Josh, Carol, and I flew into the Port-au-Prince international airport and then made our way by boat to the small island of La Gonâve just off the Haitian coast. When we arrived at our final destination, I was introduced to Da Da, our native interpreter, whom I asked about Dee Adone.

Although Da Da was initially hesitant and even evasive, I insisted on seeing my colleague's patient. As we made our way to Dee's home, the interpreter explained that our 23-year-old patient suffered not only from diabetes and tuberculosis, she probably had AIDS since she supported herself as a prostitute. With that explanation, I understood Da Da's attitude toward Dee.

When we arrived at Dee's hut, we found her lying on a small cot, the only furniture in the room. We learned that the previous dentist had bought Dee her bed and arranged to place each of the four legs in a can of water to keep ants away from her frail body. Although the woman appeared to be quite weak, I urged her to come to our makeshift clinic for the completion of her previous treatment.

When Dee showed up the following morning, I determined that she was not strong enough to withstand the extraction of all 14 remaining teeth—so I only removed eight! When I finished the extractions, Dee remained in the dental chair for a long time while I commenced treatment on another patient. After Dee finally recovered, she stumbled out of the clinic moaning softly as she went. To my dismay, I saw that this pathetic figure

was completely ignored by the other Haitians waiting for
dental care.

ate in the afternoon of the last day of our mission
tour, hundreds of patients were still waiting their
turn in line, each hoping that the extraction of one
or more teeth could ease the constant pain they
suffered. Suddenly, Carol exclaimed, "Guess who's back?"

"Who?" I asked.

"It's Dee Adone!"

Somehow, Dee had broken through the long line and fallen
exhausted onto the dental chair next to the one where I was
treating another patient. Before I could gather my thoughts,
the situation developed into a full-blown crisis. In my four
years of dental school I'd never had a class in crowd control—
much less the control of a crowd that spoke only Creole, a
language of which I was sadly ignorant.

Suddenly, a group of men began shouting, shaking their
fists at Dee Adone and—as near as I could tell from their gestures—threatening her with bodily harm. I looked to my interpreter for an explanation of what was going on, but he
remained completely silent; fear had transformed his face into
a stone mask. Then the menacing crowd began to turn on me!
Having heard terrible stories about what Haitian mobs were
capable of, I became concerned for Josh and Carol's safety.

It was at this moment I reminded myself that Josh, Carol,
and I were on this small island to do God's work—ministering
to the poor. Looking back on those events, I have no doubt
that the Lord guided my next actions since the only thing I
could rely on was the power of my faith.

Slowly, without fear, I walked past the screaming, cursing
men and made my way over to the clinic sink where I filled a
basin with water, picked up a cloth, and returned to the chair
on which Dee Adone lay. Kneeling next to my panic-stricken
patient, I removed her sandals and began washing her feet
with great care. Almost immediately, a dead silence fell over

the crowd. For the next five minutes, the only sound that filled the air was Dee Adone's rhythmic sobbing.

When I was finally satisfied with the cleansing of Dee's feet, I arose from my knees and faced the newly hushed crowd. "We have come to your island in the blessed name of Jesus Christ. Please allow us do His work in peace." Da Da, recognizing that he was no longer in danger, suddenly sprang to life and made certain his countrymen understood every word I had said.

I then removed my patient's six remaining teeth. When the treatment was completed, several men stepped forward and assisted her as she left the clinic. Many of those who, just a short time earlier, had threatened Dee Adone with angry words and bodily harm were now offering her warm smiles and their sincere compassion.

n all my life, I have never experienced a more inspiring demonstration of the Power of Faith! I will never forget it; nor will I forget Dee Adone whose misery was ended by our merciful Lord just a few years later. Since my first trip, I have returned to La Gonâve on more than a dozen missions in the hope that my tiny contribution will help reduce the awful suffering of some of God's less fortunate children—the people of Haiti. ♥

—Paul A. Bonstead, DDS

Kisses from Madagascar

he language rhythms of French and Malagasy are musical when they flow from the lips of a child. It's just another melody that becomes familiar in the towns of Madagascar. Little boys and girls are naturally close to my heart: I have reared three sons and three daughters, the parents of my 13 grandchildren.

My husband Larry and I have spent the last 20 years traveling the globe, taking his skills as a dentist into Third World nations. Indigenous people living in remote villages can live a lifetime in pain and poor health, and that's why we go to them. Larry treats their suffering. And what do I do? I sterilize instruments, hold the babies, comfort the mothers, swat the flies...and love my husband. It's teamwork, accomplished with other medical professionals who care about these people.

Our last trip took us to this island nation off the east coast of Africa. In this former French colony, the Malagasy natives are a distinctive blend of language, ethnicity, and religion. There are traces of Asian, African, and European influences. Every country I've visited has left me touched by the tenderness of the men and women we treat. But the *children*...they engrave their value on your heart. I have learned that the poor have much to give. Especially, the little ones.

Not long ago, I had to run an errand for Larry in Madagascar's southern city of Fort Dauphin. On this afternoon, it was hot and dusty, not a time to linger in the streets.

"Mademoiselle...Mademoiselle!"

I looked down to see a quartet of bright faces the color of *café au lait*: a little boy with two young sisters. The eldest girl carried a priceless package on her back: an infant sibling.

"Mademoiselle!"

I asked my interpreter what they wanted. Money... food...money *and* food?

"They want toothbrushes."

In the week since we arrived, hundreds of toothbrushes had been given to patients and visitors to our clinic. And all that these darling children (not one over the age of nine) asked for—were toothbrushes.

To the interpreter, I said, "Tell the kids to wait over there, on those steps, while I go and get a brush for each one." They scampered over and sat down in the sun. There was no shade anywhere.

Back at the clinic, I explained to Larry my welcome obligation and hurried to put together a little package for the children. My concern was the time—and the heat. I wondered if they could wait long enough for me to get back to them.

The walk into town was worrisome. Could I find them, would they still be on the steps?

I turned the corner and there they sat, little hands folded in their laps.

A matched trio of toothy grins embraced me—what a reward! I doled out an assortment of childhood joys my own children would have appreciated, so many years ago. There was a child's whistle and a toy ring for the girls, a yo-yo for the boy, and a toothbrush and toothpaste for each child. Tucked inside a dental X-ray envelope, I brought them a little expression of American sweetness: a handful of M&Ms.

I picked up one M&M and offered it to the big sister. All their smiles melted.

Their hesitancy was a jolt. Why would these children refuse this tiny morsel of goodwill?

What if you don't know it's a rare treat...what if you think it's medicine?

I took a single red droplet, put it in my mouth, and smacked my lips. *"Ummmmmmmm!"* (The international word for *delicious*.) I beamed at them, and their faces softened. Small hands reached for each of the three M&Ms I held out in my palm. They popped them in their mouths.

Facial fireworks! Those little eyes lit up like sparklers. I basked in the wonder and the light of these beautiful children.

Then the moment shattered. Three little bodies flung themselves to the pavement. And kissed my feet. Those little lips—so precious and innocent—on my dirty, dusty shoes. Three small strangers, each with a kiss. They broke my heart.

They still break my heart.

oday when I think of old lyrics and very old sonnets, each extolling *"the memory of a kiss,"* I count my kisses from Madagascar. And I give thanks...for the memory. ♥

—Elizabeth Brandenburg, DA
As told to S.G. Cooley

Saving a Life

Do what you can, with what you are, where you are.

—Theodore Roosevelt

 had been a tourist in Nepal for more than a month, camping in tents, and staying in teahouses and family lodges. One morning I was startled to hear a child crying. I suddenly realized that despite the challenging living conditions there, I had never seen or heard any children crying, not even babies—until that moment.

Curious, I followed the sound of the cries and saw a small girl in pain with her mouth wide open and several concerned adults looking in. Remembering my training, I immediately recognized that it was some kind of dental problem. I went over, took a look, and to my horror saw that several teeth were abscessed and the infection had spread into the lymph system on the child's right side. She was swollen all the way from her temple down through her armpit. I learned that she had suffered this way for over a month with only occasional complaining, simply because no one knew what to do about it. Left untreated, she would eventually die. I explained to the family that I was a "tooth doctor" and could take her to a nearby field hospital for treatment. I had already planned to visit there that very day.

Her seven-year-old sister came along for moral support. Together we made the four-hour walk up to the hospital, climbing from 11,500 to 13,000 feet on the rugged and winding two-mile high trail. During the tiring trek, I secretly hoped that the physician who worked there would be the one to take care of the tiny five-year-old because of the seriousness of her condition.

When we got to the hospital, I explained the grave situation to the physician. After he learned I was a dentist he said, "You know more about that part of the body; you'd better do it!" He called to his Sherpa assistant to bring out the "dental stuff"—a shoebox containing several pairs of pliers and a few other useless instruments all rusted together into one solid mass! The hospital had no electricity. The room was dark except for the dim light coming through a dingy corrugated plastic skylight. I was handed an unfamiliar-looking vial with mysterious foreign writing on it—supposedly filled with anesthetic— and a needle that was four inches long. I had to bend the needle into a Z-shape in order to fit it into the little girl's mouth! When she caught sight of the needle, her eyes got very big, but she didn't cry. As I injected, I prayed that this really was anesthetic, and that she wouldn't die from some toxic overdose.

The only useful instrument I had for the surgery was my Swiss Army pocketknife, a treasured gift from my father. As I pried out the infected teeth with it, the little girl trembled a few times—but still no tears. After draining as much purulence from the wound as possible, I realized there was no suture available with which to stitch it closed. So I used a wadded-up strip of cloth for her to bite on to stop the bleeding. After getting some penicillin tablets from the physician, we left.

As we walked slowly back toward the trail on the side of the mountain, I became increasingly troubled by the prospect of having to care for this child. I was worried about her survival from the infection, her weakened condition because of the crude surgery, and the probability that I would have to carry her down the steep slope back to her village. I was mostly bothered because all of this extra time would cause me to miss photographing the sunset on Mt. Everest that was only viewable from the ridge top across the valley. I could never make it down and back up the other side by dark at this rate, and I had to leave the area the next day—never to see Everest again.

hen we finally arrived at the trail edge, we could see her village almost 2,000 feet straight down below us. She immediately started running down the steep, rocky trail. As I watched her jubilant and nimble leaps toward home, I knew I could never catch her, much less keep up. Suddenly, the enormity of my selfishness hit me, and through a flood of guilty tears, I watched her deftly disappear around a corner on the endless switchbacks. I knew she had the surefootedness and commitment to make it home safely.

In that moment I learned about true courage and selflessness. I vowed I would return someday and really help out, and I did—but that's another story. She lived, and—for the first time in my life—so did I! ♥

—Sherwin R. Shinn, DDS

Dental Images

After the verb "To Love," "To Help"
is the most beautiful verb in the world.

—Bertha von Suttner

 was on a healthcare mission in Africa near the foothills of Mt. Kenya. A makeshift dental operatory had been set up for me consisting of a chair borrowed from local villagers and a bench carved out of a tree. A sugarcane fence had been constructed to keep the crowds back while they observed others being treated.

I was the only dental professional who had ever visited the area. People came for miles to have their teeth cleaned. Many had to wait a long time. I had to earn the trust of this community I was serving. Not only were dental concepts new and different, but—to them—*I* was different as well. While I struggled to work in a radically new environment, they struggled to accept me. Many were anxious about receiving treatment.

I called the name of a boy who was about seven years old. He was frightened, just like most kids his age anywhere in the world. I went over, picked him up, and sat down with him on my lap. Tears streamed down his face. In an effort to console the lad, I picked up a mirror and told him to look at those big tears. I knew he couldn't understand a word I said, but I watched as he peered curiously into the mirror. It took only a moment for me to realize that he had never seen his reflection before. The boy slowly moved his head from side to side and seemed amazed that the reflection imitated him. We both watched in the mirror as I cleaned his teeth.

The youngster left the clinic area with a big smile on his face. Not only had he survived the treatment, he had also received a lasting image of his own reflection. Wiping the tears from my eyes, I also smiled, grateful for being able to give him such a precious memory. ♥

—Cathy Milejczak, CDA, RDH, BHS

National Geographic

*Laughter is the sensation of feeling good all over
but showing it primarily in one spot.*

—Josh Billings

had been in Conakry for nearly a month when a second dental screening day was to be held at the makeshift clinic in Guinea, West Africa. Our time there was running out, and barely a dent had been made in the unremitting crowd of people seeking help. Our purpose that day was to try to screen all those interested in dental care in order to give priority to the worst cases.

Expecting a large crowd, we had arrived just before daybreak. To our surprise, nearly 300 people were already pressing in around the gates in the hope of receiving one of the few coveted dental appointments. My job, and that of three other volunteers, was to take medical histories. This proved to be a particularly challenging task. Not only were we getting everything secondhand through our interpreters, we also had to deal with the troublesome fact that few of the patients were aware of their own birthdays, let alone their medical histories.

As I proceeded with the screenings, I paid no attention to the beads of sweat that were running down my back—a common experience in West Africa. After all, the temperature was nearing the century mark, and it wasn't even noon! However when we broke for lunch I realized I couldn't continue—I had broken out in a full-blown fever. I returned to the hospital ship and didn't leave my bed for three days. I was vaguely diagnosed as having "jungle fever," the umbrella term covering everything from diarrhea to heat prostration. At least I didn't have malaria! As I lay in bed, I began to think, "Okay, I've had *enough* of Africa!" But by the end of the week I was back on my feet and returned to the clinic—drawn once again by the unending sea of desperate patients!

Our screening day was a success. We had been able to help many of those with the worst situations and pain. We even found time to squeeze in a few others as well...including a four-year-old girl whose mother had brought her to the clinic in the hope we could resolve the child's chronic oral irritation. We discovered that most of the youngster's teeth were rotten and broken, producing razor sharp edges—common symptoms that, with our limited resources, we would treat by smoothing the tooth surfaces.

"Was the child in pain?" we had the interpreter ask the mother.

To our surprise, the woman raised her shirt, showed us her bare breast capped with red teeth marks, and answered, "No, the *child* is not in pain; *I* am in pain!"

Working as a volunteer in Africa is as rewarding as it is draining. Seeing tragic and heartbreaking situations every day takes its emotional toll; there is all too little comic relief. This woman's response, flashing us with her bare breast, brought that relief. Her innocent gesture and simple statement of fact broke us up! One volunteer started laughing...then another ...and then another. The laughter was contagious. Pretty soon the mother laughed. Then the child laughed too, following her mother's example. We all stood there laughing—at what, I can't quite say, but it was good for our souls to laugh that day.

After the child was treated she left the clinic with her

mother—both their spirits lifted by our care just as their visit had lifted ours. ♥

—Julie Burton, RDH

Little Shoes

*So much has been given me, I have no time
to ponder over that which has been denied.*

—Helen Keller

ijuana, Mexico, lies just south of the border from San Diego, California. Six Saturdays a year, I—along with a female, Spanish-speaking dental assistant and my husband who lugs all our equipment and drives our truck over the rough roads—go to Tijuana to volunteer our dental services. We work alongside our medical colleagues out of a makeshift clinic in the back of a church providing minor medical and dental care.

The patients line up a few hours before our arrival to get their appointment numbers so that they can be seen in some sort of order. Late one very warm Saturday afternoon, we were relieved by the realization that we had seen all the dental patients with appointment numbers. With the heat and the sheer number of patients we had seen, my assistant and I were exhausted—ready to pack up and head on home.

At that point, the local coordinator came up to us—as she typically did at the end of the day—and asked if we could see "just one more patient."

As I often did in these highly predictable situations, I smiled and said, "Yes..." we would see "just one more patient—but *just this one very last time.*"

The little boy we saw had a minor dental problem that we quickly resolved. As I looked up to tell his mother about the procedure we had done, I noticed the baby on her lap bundled in a light blanket with his little shoes sticking out. On the bottoms of the soles were the words "Hi Mom" and "Hi Dad." I immediately recognized the shoes, and my eyes welled up with tears.

A couple of years earlier, those shoes had been gifts to my twin sons. When the boys outgrew them, I brought the shoes to Tijuana for donation to the church. My sons' names, "Matthew" and "Patrick," had been embossed on the tops of those shoes. The baby in the lap of my patient's mother had on one of each! I immediately felt an incredible sense of guilt. How selfish I had been not to want to see one more patient who needed us. Those little shoes made me realize how lucky I am to have been given so much. ♥

—Mary M. O'Connor, DDS

Flying Doctors

*Strange is our situation here upon earth. Each of us comes for a
short visit not knowing why, yet sometimes seeming to a
Divine purpose. From the standpoint of daily life, however,
there is one thing we do know: we are here for the sake
of others—for the countless unknown souls with whose fate
we are connected by a bond of sympathy.*

—Albert Einstein

he excitement of the hustling crowd of volunteers
came to an abrupt halt after an ominous phone call
warned that one of our planes—with six members
on board—may have had a bad landing near the
airport. Returning from a three-day mission in a small village
in Baja, the passengers were to join the other arrivees in
Ensenada, Mexico, at the first annual meeting of the *Los
Médicos Voladores*—LMVs or "Flying Doctors." Saturday was
to be a day of seminars and sharing of our common bond for
the more than 50 attendees who had volunteered their services
under the direction of the 26-year-old LMV organization.

The club leaders, who had been scurrying back and forth
from the quaint mission-style motel to the venue at the
mayor's office building, suddenly refocused their activities.
Everyone fell into a state of subdued shock. We ran around
hugging each other, praying it was just a hard landing and that,
somehow, all aboard were safe. Deep concern creased the face

of our club's chapter president. He rounded up several pilots, flagged a taxi, and rushed to the airport in order to assess the situation and be of whatever assistance was possible. Those who stayed at the motel paced around consoling each other, waiting for any news from the airport that was more than 15 minutes' drive away.

The missing plane was a twin-engine craft that veteran member Marv was flying. Marv, a highly competent pilot and physician, was a longtime personal friend and one of the most compassionate people I've ever met. I'd flown with him many times. Just a week earlier, he had asked me to talk to the dentist on his team, Michael, who was on his first trip. I coached Michael on what to bring and how to plan for a rewarding and fun trip. Michael had originally planned to bring his wife—also a dentist—along. However, she cancelled a few days prior to the trip after learning she was pregnant. In her place, Michael brought his assistant, Evette, also on her first trip. Another passenger on the plane was our translator, Ellen, a longtime veteran of LMV. The manifest included my dear friend, Edith, an 84-year-old, elegant, retired general practitioner devoted to women's health. Marv also had Deborah, the person responsible for bringing LMV to her hometown of San Ignacio, on board.

As the minutes ticked by, I struggled to maintain a positive attitude and told everyone all would be well. While awaiting further news, I moved away from the others, sat by myself, and reflected on my 20 years as a volunteer LMV dentist.

 learned about LMV's existence at a dental meeting and joined in a heartbeat. I immediately started planning to go on the next scheduled trip. The LMV mission statement rekindled memories of my many volunteer trips as a dentist stationed in Vietnam. Several days a month, I would join a team of volunteers, including nurses, physicians, and Red Cross personnel, on missions of mercy. We would take the Med-Evac helicopters to small, remote villages and set up primitive clinics in order to aid the orphans and the needy. The teary-eyed thanks and Velcro hugs we received from so many children and appreciative natives gave me highs and warm feelings that became very addictive. When I heard about LMV, it had been eight years since I'd experienced those feelings from which I was still suffering withdrawal symptoms. It was time to get my "fix" and renew that incredible sense of intense satisfaction. Just four weeks later, I was off to Mexico for the start of what would average out to roughly three missions a year for the next 20 years.

Los Médicos Voladores was founded in 1974 to provide free health services and education to the people of northern Mexico. The organization sends medical teams on four-day trips every month. These teams typically include a pilot, interpreter, medical professional (usually MD, dentist, or optometrist), and possibly a copilot or general volunteer. The areas we serviced were often so poor and underdeveloped that there was no dentist within a day's drive. When I first joined LMV, some towns we served had no telephones. We simply announced our arrival by flying circles low over the town before landing our small planes on the community's dirt strip. Then someone would drive around town with a loudspeaker so that people would know we were there to help. The next day, before we even opened our clinic, the villagers would be lined up at the door.

On every trip, I get hugs and sincere thanks that fill my heart to the brim. On my first trip, the town elementary school teacher came in with a broken off front tooth; she was a pretty young lady who, for five years, had had a spoiled smile. I repaired the tooth and filled in the gap. After looking in the mirror, she wept with joy. She hugged me, kissed me on the cheek, blessed me with the sign of the cross, and said that I was surely an angel from Heaven.

For years my daughter, Tiffany, saw the sparkle in my eye when I returned from these trips and begged to go. When she turned 14, she took Spanish in high school, learned to dental assist, and has come with me once a year for the past seven years. Since dental assisting is not her chosen career, I ask before each trip why she continues to volunteer for these missions. She simply shrugs and says, "I do it for numerous reasons, but—most of all—I just love helping people and seeing their grateful smiles."

My reverie ended abruptly when I heard the Ensenada reception desk phone ring. The clerk handed the phone to Kathleen, our trip co-coordinator. Moments later, she went white. The plane had crashed short of the runway, and all six of our friends were dead! Shock, disbelief, and emotional turmoil swept over the members.

The chairman of the club, Tom, returned from the crash site, gathered us around, and outlined a course of action needed. Despite the incredible grief, we all decided to continue the seminar and dedicate it to the memory of our comrades. Committees were formed to deal with the necessary duties in this type of tragedy. The Mexican officials turned their offices over to us, and we carried on.

There is always risk in flying small airplanes to remote areas of Mexico. There is risk in driving there as well. Every last member agreed that these risks were worth the tremendous rewards and the good that we do in Mexico. Ironically, the wrenching sense of loss that the death of our comrades had produced empowered us to greater achievements over the next few months. Our club grew by leaps and bounds; and our relationship with the Mexican government became more productive.

e all have our own reasons for serving as volunteers. Our friends had now given their lives for their reasons. They may have done it just to be philanthropic, or like me, they may have given of themselves for selfish reasons. I do it for the adventure of setting up a modern dental clinic in remote places that sometimes have dirt floors and no electricity. I do it for the warm and wonderful feeling of satisfaction and happiness that engulfs me for months after my Flying Doctor trips. I do it because I love it—and I always will! ❤

—Adrian D. Fenderson, DDS

6

GOLDEN YEARS

The tide recedes but leaves behind
bright seashells on the sand;
The sun goes down but gentle warmth
still lingers on the land;
The music stops and echoes on
in soft and sweet refrains;
For every joy that passes,
something beautiful remains.

—Anonymous

Keepsake Crown

avid and his family became patients of mine about
1963 shortly after I opened my dental practice in
London. He owned a well-known and successful
Jewish delicatessen. Whenever my wife and I
passed his shop, we stopped in to enjoy his warm joviality and
stock up on his collection of unique and hard-to-find
Continental foods.

David had a gold crown on his upper left second premolar
and, long before the start of his visits to my surgery—the
British term for what you Americans call a "dental office"—
this tooth was compromised due to gum disease. It quickly
became apparent that there was something special about this
crowned tooth because, during his regular teeth cleaning
appointments, David only wanted it scaled gently rather than
receiving a more aggressive treatment.

After some years I found out more about David and his
background. He was a Pole, and around the start of World
War II he had been captured and forced to fight as a Russian
soldier. When his part of Poland was overrun, he lost everything he possessed with one small exception—a single gold
crown that had been made just before the war. In 1975, this
tooth started to develop an abscess and—after much soul
searching by the patient—it was agreed that extraction was the
only option. David was extremely upset about losing the tooth
from his mouth, but he would still be able to have it as a keep-

sake. "I can't tell you how much I'm going to miss seeing that crown in the mirror when I shave in the morning," he told me with a sad wistfulness.

The day I removed the tooth I made some excuse that the infected root should be sterilized before I gave it back to him, and I kept it in my surgery. Some weeks later, David came in for the bridge preparation and impressions. I showed him his old crown and root but told him I needed the tooth to "measure up the correct shape" for the fixed bridge being made to fill the new gap in his dentition.

Back in the laboratory, I asked my technician to construct a three-unit bridge. The first premolar in front of the gap and the molar behind the gap were conventional bonded porcelain-to-gold units. But in the center, a "dummy" had to be made where the old tooth and crown had been. At this point I cut the root away from under the old Polish gold crown. My technician was then able to mount and cement the keepsake crown in the "dummy" space. The final effect was just as though the old gold tooth had always been between the two newly crowned teeth.

At the fitting stage, I managed to avoid showing David the bridge while I set it firmly in place. I then announced that he could look at his new teeth. Slowly and deliberately handing him a mirror, I asked if he would like his keepsake crown back. "Oh, yes. I want it very much, please."

"You already have it, David. It's right back where it belongs." I told him what had been done, and with every syllable spoken, I watched as an old soldier surrendered to his tears.

t is rare for a patient to break down and sob with pleasure in the surgery. As I realized that David was now in his mid-seventies, I worried for a few moments that I might have precipitated a medical crisis. Fortunately, he quickly recovered his composure and consented to having the bridge cemented in place. A few

minutes later, David left the surgery wearing a broad smile I'd
never seen before. His tearful happy face is a memory I will
always cherish. ❤

—John McCormack, DDS

The Colonel

Age is a question of mind over matter.
If you don't mind,
it doesn't matter.

—Satchel Paige

he Colonel is one of my favorite patients. I first met him 12 years ago when he was 81. By then, it seemed he had already lived two lifetimes. Two wars. Two wives—with each marriage lasting more than 30 years. And finally, a new career as a teacher-writer-raconteur.

In my 33 years as a dental hygienist, I've also lived two lifetimes. I measure my years in people rather than calendar pages. After working with thousands of patients, I'm well into the second generation of many families. In our memories, there are always a distinguished few characters who stand out, and among the notable people in my life, there will always be the Colonel.

The Colonel's impact on me was immediate. He had the energy of a man half his age, getting up each morning to do calisthenics and fly the American flag. He is completely bald—Yul Brynner style—and it isn't hard to envision him in the musical *The King and I,* dancing with Deborah Kerr in her satin ball gown. Almost anything will trigger a story from the Colonel, delivered with rapid-fire speech and tinged with his wonderful humor. We learned to extend the office schedule

for him since we always succumb to his charm—and lose
all track of time.

The Colonel's smile today is beautiful. A few lost teeth
have been replaced with fixed bridges. In his ninth decade, he
chose to have us place crowns on the front teeth. That gave
him a handsome grin in which he takes delight! He follows
each dental visit with a letter. Pounded out on an old manual
typewriter, each missive is sprinkled with underlined words
and *exclamation marks!* Around the margins are handwritten
comments, last-minute thoughts he can't resist adding. These
are notes thanking us for our care, often touching on national
and international news of the day. And he always includes a
comment about the wonder of being able to keep his teeth for
so many years.

everal years ago, the Colonel developed health
problems that took him to the local VA hospital.
When we routinely ask about his health during
dental examinations, he gives us a military brief-
ing on his most recent concerns, treating them like mere incon-
veniences in his busy schedule. But the story he always
reports is that at each hospital visit he is approached by a
nurse bearing a container who says, "Now Colonel, please put
your teeth in here."

He replies, "Sorry, ma'am—I can't do that."

The nurse—perhaps accustomed to a more disagreeable or
disoriented patient—invariably insists, "Now Colonel, you
know you have to take your teeth out! Put them in here!"

At this point in the little hospital drama, he answers,
"Young lady, these teeth are firmly attached. If you think
you can get them out, you just try!" And he watches with
amusement while nurses and doctors crowd around to see
his wonderful teeth. Little does the hospital staff know that
their reactions will provide raw material for the Colonel's
next story. I'm absolutely convinced his storytelling is a vital
element in keeping him alert and irresistibly charming.

I have no doubt that he'll live to be 100. And when the Colonel meets his Maker, he'll report to the gates with a snap of his salute—and a world-class smile. ♥

—Sue O'Brien, RDH

Fish Story

*If people ever finally figure out what's important in life,
there's gonna be a shortage of fishin' poles.*

—Sign on a Northwoods bait shop

 wizened and wrinkled little old man in worn overalls—not *old*, actually, *ancient* would be a better word—appeared at the front desk and announced that he had come to get him some "store-bought teeth." Of course they had to be the brightest and whitest that money could buy. Though it was obvious the man didn't have a lot of material possessions, he pulled a wad of hundred-dollar bills out of his bib pocket and proudly stated that he could pay—he'd been saving for years to be able to have new teeth.

In the course of his treatment, the new patient and the Doc became big buddies through their common love of fishing. As each tried to top the other's story of "the one that got away," our entire staff came to look forward to these visits. By the time he had visited the office a half dozen times, the old fella' had earned a soft spot in our hearts. Finally, with new dentures in place, he left our office with a beaming new smile and a lightness in his step that I hadn't seen before.

A few weeks later, our friend returned—chin on chest and toothless.

It seems that the big one, the *REALLY* big one, finally

didn't get away; and in his excitement, the old man had spit his dentures into the lake! He was ready to start saving all over again.

As one fisherman to another, our doctor took care of his needs—gratis of course—and the old fella' once again left with a smile on his deeply wrinkled face. Observing all of this, it seems I've developed a new appreciation for small acts of kindness and avid fishermen. ❤

—Leanne Haynes, RDH, BS

Questionnaire

n elderly gentleman was escorted into my office seeking relief from a painful tooth. Since he was a new patient, I sat next to him and began to review his health history questionnaire. I did this out of deference to the patient's age, as well as to determine the reason why he had indicated "yes" to having AIDS.

When asked if he did, in fact, have AIDS, the old gentleman's words were staccato-like and *loudly* indignant, "Yeah, I got 'em, but they ain't working so good! Must need new batteries." ♥

—Gregory R. Johnson, DDS

Curing Cancer

The greater part of our happiness
or misery depends on
our mental disposition
and not on our circumstances.

—Martha Washington

er name was Mildred, and she was probably the oldest person I had ever met. The tiny little lady lowered herself heavily, deliberately into my dental chair. History was etched in her face. She was ladylike, almost prim, as she painstakingly arranged herself. Then she looked up. Instantly my attention was redirected. The tears in her pale blue eyes made me forget her age. Sensing her need for confidence, I closed the door and asked what was wrong.

Mildred wasn't one of my established patients. It was a stretch, in fact, to call *any* of my patients established. It was 1964, and I was just 25 years old—a brand-new dentist. Most of my patients hadn't been with me long enough to return for a six-month checkup!

She hesitated before responding—taking a couple of shallow breaths—before deciding to answer. "I'm...dying," she stammered. "I'm dying of mouth cancer. And I want you to tell me how long I have before I....." She paused, then whispered, "How long do I have to live?"

She was 84 years old, her chart said. Back in the sixties, 84 was ancient. People just didn't live as long then as they do now. In those days, 65 was old, 70 was very old, and 75 was really, really old. You just didn't meet people in their eighties. But, in spite of her extreme age, Mildred wasn't ready to die. She wanted to *live!*

"Mouth cancer?" I repeated and asked her to let me take a look.

She'd been wearing dentures—a full set—for 35 years, she told me.

The affected area became apparent as soon as I removed the dentures. The gum around the upper right wisdom tooth was inflamed and angry looking. Her dentures had been rubbing the area, exacerbating the existing inflammation. I could readily appreciate how uncomfortable she must have been. I studied the area closely, careful not to comment until I was absolutely sure. What I found was surprising— but not dangerous.

The inflamed area did look painful—even alarming—but it was nothing that would kill her. In fact, it was not a typical ailment for an elderly woman but rather something most dentists find in their younger patients—their *much* younger patients. But was I positive? I inspected the area again to make sure there was no mistake. No, this definitely was not cancer!

"Ma'm," I said, smiling, "I have good news." Mildred's eyes widened. "You don't have cancer," I said.

"I don't?" she asked hopefully.

"No," I said, "you definitely do *not* have cancer."

"Then what is it? What is wrong with me?" she asked.

"Absolutely nothing is wrong with you," I said. "You're just teething." She was actually cutting a wisdom tooth!

With that news, Mildred threw her head back and laughed out loud with relief. I removed the culprit—a simple procedure, as the tooth was small and underdeveloped—in no time. I almost could have taken it out with my fingers.

hen it was all over, that prim old lady who had entered the operatory with such deliberate heaviness practically skipped out of my office—and I never saw her again! I don't know how much longer she lived, but one thing I feel sure of is this: no matter what end she faced, she didn't die from mouth cancer. ♥

—Clyde T. Padgett, Jr., DDS

Full-Service Station

It takes so little to make people happy—just a touch,
if we know how to give it, just a word fitly spoken,
or a slight readjustment of some bolt or pin or bearing
in the delicate machinery of a human soul.

—Frank Crane

he nursing home van pulled into our parking lot. Shortly afterward, my 89-year-old dental patient slowly shuffled into the operatory. "Hi Eva, how are you feeling today?" I asked.

"Been better," she snapped, as she gingerly lowered herself into the chair.

When Eva handed over her upper denture, I noticed that her gums were red and swollen. "You really need to get some air to your gums and massage them a little. Are you remembering to take your denture out at night?"

"Can't do that. They'll steal 'em. They stole Myra's denture, you know. They've been stealing my hard candy too! My mouth gets real dry and I need my hard candies. I have to sleep with my candy jar under my pillow now. They won't be getting their hands on my candy anymore and they're sure not getting their hands on my teeth!"

"Well maybe you can keep your denture under your pillow at night, right next to your candy jar."

"Might get a little lumpy," she sighed, "but I guess I'll

give it a try."

Since Eva had only six lower front teeth remaining, it didn't take long for me to complete her cleaning. I pushed the tray back and sat her up a bit, "Now we just need to wait for the doctor to come in and check on your teeth."

"That's fine, I got no place to go," she said, and then began to tell me all about her family and life in the nursing home. When she spoke about her family, she seemed to soften...her defenses slipping away. "My daughter used to come by every week and brush my hair. I always looked forward to her visits," she said, her eyes welling up with tears. "Now she's too busy with the grandchildren, running them all over the place. She used to read to me; I really miss that. She'd even clip these unsightly hairs off of my chin. No one will clip them off in the nursing home. Nobody will do that for me anymore," she said with quivering lips.

I had a hard time containing my emotions as I watched her tears threaten to spill over. I also had to struggle to keep my eyes off of her long, curly, white chin hairs.

"I'll be right back," I assured her and hurried out of the room. Soon I returned, armed with a pair of suture scissors. "Would you like me to take care of them for you?" I asked. "Your chin hairs—would you like me to cut them back?"

The tears then rolled down her cheeks. "Would you really do that for me? Bless you, honey."

"This is a full-service dental office. We like to see *all* our patients leave here with big smiles. I'd be happy to help you out." With scissors in hand, I aimed my dental light at her chin. "Now sit still and this won't hurt a bit," I told her.

As I clipped off the final hair, I heard footsteps behind me that came to an abrupt halt. I turned around to see the dentist, staring at the sight, red-faced with his mouth hanging open. Tossing the chin hairs and my gloves into the trash, I explained the situation to my flabbergasted boss. "I told Eva we were a full-service dental office; and she decided to go for the complete treatment. I believe she's ready for you to check her teeth now!"

We both turned and looked at Eva. Her nearly toothless smile brightened the room. ❤

—Nancy Roe-Pimm, RDH

Sweet Surrender

*Careful grooming may take 20 years off a woman's age,
but you can't fool a long flight of stairs.*

—Marlene Dietrich

 ilith, an eccentric Manhattan socialite, has her teeth cleaned every three months in our periodontal practice. Her lower arch—in dentistry, we call jaws "arches"—consists of implants only—no natural teeth. Her upper arch—called the maxillary arch—has no teeth at all since she lacks sufficient bone to support implants. Her only alternative is to wear an upper denture. "Horrible!" she says whenever she refers to her "condition."

Well into her seventies, Lilith appears better preserved than a jar of peaches. Her body still maintains the build of a lean teen; her attire and hairstyle are totally hip. She prides herself on her appearance and has sworn never, *ever,* to reveal the truth about her man-made top teeth. Lilith's friends are in constant awe of her maintenance magic and always consult her regarding diet, vitamins, exercise, cosmetics, fashion, restaurants, fortune-tellers, doctors, dentists, etc.

Recently, Lilith referred her close friend, Dottie, to our office. Dottie is also a very attractive woman in her seventies, though not quite as eccentric as her friend. However, Dottie's lovely appearance was immediately downgraded when she opened her mouth—revealing a set of discolored, worn—but *natural*—upper teeth. Aware of the unsightliness of her stained and stubby dentition, she wanted to enhance her appearance and insisted that her teeth resemble those of her friend, Lilith. Naturally this led our office to refer her to the prosthodontist Lilith used, still never revealing the hidden truth of Lilith's maxillary arch. Dottie took our lead, and her teeth turned out beautifully—both technically and cosmetically. She looked wonderful, and the luster in her pale blue eyes was made even more effervescent by the enhancement of her new crowns. Of course this made me quite happy and pleased since I felt partly responsible for such a positive result. Therefore I cannot tell you how stunned I was when Dottie tearfully expressed how devastated she felt. She worried that her teeth did *not* resemble Lilith's at all. As I tried to console her by explaining how each person's dentition is different, I couldn't help but think to myself, *if she only knew!*

If only Dottie could see the humiliation and frustration Lilith experiences each and every time she comes to our office and has to remove her denture; and the fear she has that someone might see her in my operatory "naked"—without her denture. Lilith's artificial apparatus is a constant reminder that she cannot regain her youth, despite her extraordinarily well-preserved appearance.

What I find most interesting about this situation is Lilith's compassion and sense of humor. When Dottie finally told Lilith of her disappointment, Lilith keenly felt her friend's pain and was unable to keep her secret any longer. She simply removed her denture, handed it to Dottie, and said, "Here, you want it? It's yours. After all, what are friends for?" ❤

—Robin Brenner, RDH

Sharing

*I knew we would get married
when we started talking about
what it would be like to grow old together.*

—Joanna Dobbs

he Johnsons were a sweet, adorable couple in their eighties. I had been their dentist for more than a decade and had watched them lean more and more on each other as the years passed. I especially noticed the way they would grasp one another's hands a bit tighter as they walked a more aged path.

The Johnsons were inseparable, never one without the other. Like many couples that have passed the half-century mark of togetherness, the Johnsons had even begun to look somewhat alike. One's frail hands, tottering step, and bent posture seemed mirrored in the other's.

I saw the Johnsons professionally only occasionally because they both wore full dentures. One spring morning, they visited my office to have Mrs. Johnson's dentures adjusted.

"They hurt her real bad," said Mr. Johnson. "Probably need whittlin' on."

I took a quick look at the dentures as I removed them from her mouth. "How are *your* teeth doing, Mr. Johnson?" I inquired.

"Not bad," he responded. "Feel a bit tight, though."

"Mind if I look at them?" I asked.

As I took both sets of dentures back to the lab to examine them more closely, my initial suspicions were confirmed. The Johnsons had somehow—somewhere along the way—gotten their lower dentures mixed up. She had his; he had hers! I cleaned up the dentures and delivered each set to its proper mouth. In return, I received exclamations of joy and thanks.

"No charge, Mr. Johnson. I hope they feel much better."

"What'd you do?"

"Not much, really. Have a good day!"

As they gingerly leaned on each other with clasped hands and shuffled toward the door, I felt a warm tear well up in my eye. The bonds of love and familiarity know no bounds. ❤

—Robert F. Weed, DDS

My Valentine

*Unable are the loved to die,
for love is immortality.*

—Emily Dickinson

he first time Mr. and Mrs. Sinclair came into our office, I was deeply moved by this man's love for his wife. He called her "my Valentine." I observed that Mrs. Sinclair walked a little slowly, although she managed quite well while I cleaned her teeth. When it was time to leave, Mr. Sinclair said, "Let's go, Valley." It took me a moment to realize that "Valley" was his nickname for "my Valentine."

At their recall appointments six months later, Mrs. Sinclair moved very slowly and didn't talk much. That was okay because Mr. Sinclair kept up the chatter during both their procedures. He explained that his Valentine was tiring more easily now, but that he was going to take good care of her. He assured me she would be just fine. They left the office holding hands.

Mr. Sinclair and his Valentine returned six months later, and to my surprise, Valley was in a wheelchair. It was obvious she was deteriorating both mentally and physically; but Mr. Sinclair was, as always, devoted and optimistic. He let me know that the doctors said Valley had Alzheimer's, but he would be there to help her "all the way." During each visit, he shared with me the joys and triumphs of caring for his wife. He took great pride in attending to her needs because she'd always been supportive of him in the years when she had been healthy. He told me how he helped her wash and dress; he even brushed her teeth. For that visit, Valley required only a little assistance while getting out of her wheelchair and into my patient chair.

At their next appointments, Mrs. Sinclair had more difficulty moving around, so I cleaned her teeth while she sat in the wheelchair. Mr. Sinclair patted her hands and reassured her during the entire procedure. Mrs. Sinclair responded with a few grunts, but there was no verbalization. As usual, Mr. Sinclair was upbeat and stressed that Valley had some really good days and would be getting better real soon. He always told me what he had fed her for breakfast and how well she had eaten. From time to time during the procedure, he rubbed her cheek and called her "my Valentine."

Mr. Sinclair arrived alone for his next visit. He said Valley wasn't up to coming in anymore; he had a neighbor sitting with her while he was gone. He took pride in telling me that Valley's eyes would still light up when she saw him. He knew she loved him and would have cared for him just as attentively if their roles had been reversed. But, for now, he did everything for her. He bathed, dressed, and fed her; though he confided he found it easier to leave Valley in her nightgown than dress her, so that's what he did. He explained that his wife didn't sleep well, so he'd have to get up several times each night. But he didn't mind; he was happy to be there for his beloved Valley.

he next time I saw Mr. Sinclair, he told me right away, "The Good Lord has taken my Valentine to Heaven, and one day I'm going to join her." He told me not to be sad, though. He was happy he'd been able to know and love someone as special as the woman he called "my Valentine." ♥

—Mary S. Pelletier, RDH, BS

Song of Love

How do I love thee? Let me count the ways.
I love thee with the breath, smiles, tears, of all my life.

—Elizabeth Barrett Browning

ur office is a single-dentist practice. However, we have an arrangement with a semi-retired dentist who helps out one day a week when he sees five or six patients. Since he only works on dentures and partials, he primarily sees our older patients.

Occasionally, our "special" doctor makes house calls to see patients unable to travel. I remember one man who sought dental care for his invalid wife. After going to the patient's home to conduct a preliminary examination, our doctor felt the need to have her moved into the office. There, he would have access to the special equipment necessary to deal with her pain.

The husband arranged to have his wife brought over by ambulance. As the paramedics wheeled her in, I saw before me a slender, itty-bitty thing—a woman obviously dying and in great pain. Her fear of the office was so great I could actually "feel" it. It was on that day the most magical thing I've ever experienced happened before my eyes and ears.

Hovering next to the patient's gurney was this incredible man who gently held her hand while singing an exquisitely beautiful and soothing song. The world—as I had known it up until that moment—changed forever.

In my career, I have witnessed several divorces due to sickness. The healthy spouses simply didn't have the commitment to stand by their mates "in *sickness* and in health." But that day I witnessed a man still loving and caring for his beloved wife to the very end. She soon adjusted to the office atmosphere, and the doctor began to work on her. During the entire procedure, the patient's husband never left her side. Nor did he stop singing his exquisite, soothing song.

Who were they? I can't remember.

How long ago did this happen? I have no idea.

What was she dying of? I haven't a clue.

Who referred them to us? A little angel who knew that I needed to see true love for what it really is.

What was the name of the song? I don't know—but I'm sure she still hears it even if she's no longer among the living. ♥

—Mary Jo Pletz, RDH

7

LITTLE SURPRISES

*If you could choose
one characteristic
to get you through life,
choose a sense of humor.*

—Jennifer James

Expensive Diet

ennifer, my four year old daughter, sat on the bathroom counter as usual while I started the bedtime countdown by brushing her teeth. Later, I would tuck her under the covers, read her a story, join her in prayer, and give her a goodnight kiss.

On that evening, however, Jennifer said it was only fair she should get the chance to brush my teeth when I was done with hers. That sounded fine to me; so when I finished, I handed her my brush, and she started the reciprocal treatment.

Now before I continue, you must understand that most of my molars have gold fillings, inlays, or crowns. After a short while, Jennifer stopped, looked carefully inside my mouth, and asked, "Daddy, have you been eating Mommy's jewelry?" ❤

—Stanley J. Larsen, DDS
(1952–2001)

Wasted Effort

have the pleasure of serving three generations of one family in my practice. They are all on periodic scheduling and visit the office regularly. Without exception, the members of this family are a joy to know and work with.

On one occasion, I had the grandfather booked for a filling. As it turned out, he brought his granddaughter with him since he was babysitting her for the day. While I worked on the elderly gentleman, the little girl sat with us in the operatory and seemed to be waiting with some anticipation. When Grandpa's filling was completed, I began to say my goodbyes to both visitors.

Instead of accompanying her grandfather out of the operatory, the child climbed into the dental chair as if she were expecting me to treat her. I then realized she thought she had come to the office for her own appointment. I explained that this visit was solely for her grandfather and that she did not require any dental treatment.

Upon hearing this news, the girl seemed more than a little disappointed—not the usual response when someone is freed from seeing the dentist! I asked the youngster what was wrong. She looked at me in the way only an innocent child can, and asked, "Do you mean I brushed my teeth today for nothing?" ♥

—Ira Marder, DDS, FAGD

Family Dentistry

 even-year-old Jimmy was sitting in my chair scheduled for extraction of an upper front tooth and
sporting a shiner on his right eye. "Hi, Jimmy, what
happened to your eye?" I asked.

"My sister," he replied sullenly.

"Boy, she must have been mad at you."

"Naw, she was just trying to help me pull my tooth."

"So how did she black your eye pulling your tooth?"

"She tied a long piece of floss to my tooth and the other
end to a doorknob. I had to wait a long time; and when my dad
finally came through the door, my dumb sister had put me on
the wrong side!"

Jimmy let me know in no uncertain terms he would never
let his sister do any more dental work for him. ❤

—Harry T. Keyes, DDS

Soft Diet

*Live in such a way that you would not be worried about
selling your parrot to the town gossip.*

—Will Rogers

y dad, who was also a dentist, loved to tell about a patient who returned to the office with an unusual problem several days after receiving a new denture. In front of his four-year-old son—whom he had brought along as an observer—the patient unfolded a handkerchief and displayed the denture with several of the front teeth broken out. Projecting great indignation, the patient inquired, "Well, Doc, what are you going to do about fixing my new denture? Obviously, it must have been defective to have broken so easily."

My dad then asked, "Tell me, just how did this happen?"

The patient replied, "I just bit into a sandwich, and the teeth came out."

The man's young son—ever ready to help out with the story and not at all shy—then spoke up, *"But Daddy, don't you remember? You broke your teeth when you tried to take the cap off your beer bottle!"* ❤

—Robert E. Riddle, DDS

Marital Status

 once had a three-year-old girl come in for her first visit. She was so cute with her curly blond hair that you just wanted to hug her. So I asked if she was married.

"No," was her reply.

"Why not?"

" 'Cause I'm not old enough, silly!"

"Will you marry me when you grow up?"

"No."

"Why not?"

Hands on her hips, exasperation written all over her face, she said, " 'Cause you'll be *dead!*"

I never asked that question again. ❤

—Mohamed Hussein, DDS

Shhhhhhhhh!

 hen I first started practicing dentistry, a very bright and intelligent woman who taught ancient Greek at one of the country's leading universities brought her precocious daughter in for some necessary dental work. With a scholar for a mother and a lawyer for a father, this was one smart child. Unlike so many of my patients, this girl was comfortable, unafraid, and, frankly, quite fascinated by what we were going to do. The procedure to be performed involved two restorations—fillings—with local anesthesia.

Most youngsters—and adults, for that matter—fear the needle, hate the injection, exaggerate the anticipated pain, deplore the numb lips or tongue, etc., so I was worried about my ability to take care of this child's needs and still keep her confidence. I also wanted to remove any possibility she would be fearful of returning for future treatment. Then I reminded myself about what I was taught in dental school: "Tell-Show-Do." I simply explained the procedure, showed her the cavity with the aid of a small mirror, and administered the anesthetic.

Everything went well. When I finally pulled the needle out, to break the ice and to prevent the inevitable crying, I quickly raised my index finger to my lips and whispered: "Shhhhhhhhh! Don't talk loud; your tooth is asleep!"

In response, she tilted her head, looked at me with big brown eyes, shrugged, smiled, and said, "Oh, yes, I can hear them snoring." ❤

—Robert Reyto, DDS, FAACD

Bloodcurdling Screams

I know you're highly recommended, but I really don't know what you can possibly do," insisted Rachel's mother.

The blond-haired, blue-eyed, freckle-faced six-year-old did not look so tough. Her mother was telling me that four previous dentists had tried unsuccessfully to fill her daughter's two cavities. "None of them could get anywhere at all," she related, "and they practically threw us out of their offices! They said I have no choice but to take Rachel for general anesthesia."

I was never one to shrink from a difficult task. My mind recoiled at the thought of subjecting this child to the potential dangers of a general anesthetic. A difficult patient? Ha! I hadn't yet met a pediatric patient I couldn't manage. I saw this child as a challenge I could not resist. And, besides, she looked so positively angelic!

I told the mother that I'd like to try and would appreciate it if she would sit near the child in the dental operatory during treatment.

"Okay," she sighed, "but I'm warning you, my daughter is absolutely unmanageable!"

I seated the child, and with great verbal and digital dexterity, charmed my way through administering an injection of local anesthetic. As soon as Rachel realized she was getting numb, she began screaming.

Bloodcurdling screams. Wave after wave of ear splitting, bloodcurdling screams, without letup. The child inhaled and screamed, inhaled and screamed, inhaled and screamed. I had seen it all before, and waited a few moments for the child to exhaust herself. Five minutes passed, ten minutes passed; I admired the child's stamina.

The mother began to look concerned. I winked and nodded reassuringly. While I sat behind and to the right of the supine patient, Ronnie, a brand-new dental assistant, sat on the patient's left, and Rina, a more experienced assistant, sat near the child's legs, attempting to restrain their wild kicking.

"What's Dr. Galler going to do?" whispered the very pale and shaken new assistant. "Don't worry," soothed Rina, "he's very good with kids. He'll know what to do." I noticed, however, that her left eyebrow was arched and her lips were set in a grim, straight line.

Meanwhile, the child continued to inhale and scream, inhale and scream. I tried every trick in my repertoire. I tried the Tell-Show-Do technique. I held up her wrist and demonstrated. "See, Mr. Tickle Tooth is going to wash all the dirt out of your tooth, and Mr. Thirsty here is going to vacuum up all the dirt and water." The dramatic, bloodcurdling screams intensified; inhale and scream, inhale and scream. I noticed that the receptionist raised the volume of the office's elevator music and closed the door to my treatment room tightly.

I leaned close to the child's ear and whispered, "I know why you're crying. You're crying because you're afraid. But, once you see how easy it is to clean your teeth, you'll never have to cry or be scared of the dentist again."

No effect, the screaming continued.

I warned her that if she continued to scream, her mother would have to leave the room and wait outside. No success.

I sent the very apprehensive mother out of the room. There was no discernible letup in the screams. My receptionist came in and whispered that if I was trying to empty out our waiting room, I was doing a pretty good job of it.

I tried intimidation. Bribery. Pleading. Logic. Threats. I tried physical restraints. Nothing. The screaming continued unabated. It was cool in the room, but my forehead was covered with perspiration.

I was exhausted and at my wits' end. Suddenly, inspiration struck me. "Okay, Rachel," I announced, "I'm going to clean your tooth now, and I want you to scream as loud as you can, and kick your feet as hard as you can!"

The child turned to me suddenly and said, "Huh?"

"That's right," I continued, "Please. I need you to scream very, very loud now while I clean your tooth."

Rachel folded her arms defiantly and pouted, "No! I will not!" A warm glow passed over me. I grabbed my instruments and dove into the tooth. My assistant suctioned as I cleaned and shaped the cavity, all the while urging the child to please, please scream, cry, and kick.

"No, no, I won't," insisted the stubborn child, through cotton rolls and numb lips. I invited the mother back into the room. She looked stunned as I continually implored the child to scream, while my assistant and I worked at super-fast motion, and the child refused to utter a single sound. I completed the procedure. The mother stared in disbelief at her daughter.

"Now, Rachel," I begged, as I pulled off my gloves triumphantly, "please promise me that when you come next week for your other filling, you'll scream loudly and kick your feet up and down."

"No," insisted the child, "I'm not going to make any noise, no matter what you want!"

I strode out of the room as the assistants and mother stared at me with their mouths wide open. For the rest of the day, I was like a god to my staff. ❤

—Jeffrey M. Galler, DDS, MAGD

Easy Choice

arly in my career as a dental practice management consultant, I spent a memorable morning in the operatory of an oral surgeon. I'll simply refer to him as Dr. Foster. Squirming in the patient's chair was a very frightened eight-year-old.

Wearing a smart new business suit, I gripped my clipboard and pen, intent on documenting the proceedings. This excerpt of that 20-year-old report—from memory, of course—is repeated here solely for your reading pleasure.

—Warning—

*What follows is not intended as
a recommendation for pediatric care!*

Robbie was scared to death. In considerable pain with a mouthful of abscessed primary teeth, he desperately needed the services of an oral surgeon. In order to begin the two-hour restoration, injections of anesthetic were required.

The sight of a small syringe tipped with a slender, inch-long needle sent Robbie into a fit. He cowered in the chair, screaming, while his little arms and legs flailed about in wild gyrations. Sensitive to his patient's distress, the oral surgeon handed the offending instrument to his assistant. The syringe was retired to the counter while Robbie slumped into exhaustion.

As a first-time observer of such violent patient behavior, I was stunned. And I wondered how Dr. Foster could possibly proceed.

He gave a knowing nod to his assistant. With swift precision, she produced a covered, stainless steel tray and set it in front of the child.

Dr. Foster patted the towel draped over the tray. *"Robbie, in order for us to make your mouth stop hurting, I'm going to have to put some sleepy medicine next to your teeth. The instrument I use to squirt the medicine is called a 'syringe.' I could use your advice about this. Now, Robbie, you tell me: Which one do you want me to use?"* And he lifted the towel, revealing...

A foot-long, one-inch-diameter horse syringe tipped with a blunt, three-inch needle. Next to the veterinary injector lay— in all its newfound delicacy—a standard syringe.

"I'll take *that* one, the *little* one! The *lit-tle* one!"

In no time at all, the anesthetic was administered and Robbie's successful surgery was completed without further interruption. ♥

—Linda L. Miles, CSP, CMC

Cutting Confusion

om, our newest patient, was the most sophisticated eight-year-old I'd ever met "up close and personal." Dressed in a suit, white shirt, and tie—topped off with a pair of horn-rimmed glasses—he looked like a miniature adult. I could tell by the way his parents behaved that this boy was pushed hard to do well and excel. I sort of felt sorry for the little guy.

I brought the boy back to my chair and began looking at his teeth. After a preliminary exam, I said, "Tom, it looks like you may need braces one of these days."

I wasn't trying to make him angry, but he threw his arms into the air and exclaimed, "Oh, that's just *great!*"

"What's the matter, Tom?" I asked.

"Nothing special, I'm just stressed out," he replied.

I thought to myself, *"My goodness, what does an eight-year-old have to be stressed out about? Poor guy."* I asked, "What are you so stressed out about?"

"Well," Tom answered, "I have two papers due for school, my parents told me I need a vasectomy, and now you're telling me I need braces!"

"What?" I asked myself. *"He needs a vasectomy? That just doesn't make sense."* I wasn't sure if I should ask or not, but I decided to take the risk. "Tom, do you know what a vasectomy is?"

"Of course I do," the boy replied defensively.

"Well, tell me."

In response, Tom lifted his upper lip revealing that thin piece of pink tissue—known as the *frenum*—attached to the gum and lip. "I have to have this cut."

"Oh," I thought laughing to myself, "what Tom needed was to have his frenum cut, a procedure known as a *frenectomy.*"

At that point, I decided it wasn't my place to explain to my young patient the difference between a *frenectomy* and a *vasectomy*—I'd leave that to his parents. I have no idea how many people Tom had told that he needs a vasectomy, but I hope someone teaches him what it really means before he gets married! Needless to say, that little guy made my day! ❤

—David Zamboni, RDH, BS

Shattered Confidence

s I came to the entrance of the operatory to request an examination of my hygiene patient, the doctor had just finished giving an injection to a nine-year-old boy. "Okay, this time we're going to do the right side," he said.

Upon hearing that, the lad bolted upright and—with serious concern—asked, "Does that mean the last time we did the *wrong* side?" ❤

—Linda Williams, RDH

Survival Instinct

he instinct for survival is apparent at an early age, as is easily demonstrated by an episode that occurred in my dental office.

Anticipating my own surgery, I mentioned to the parent of one of my patients that I would be out for a couple of weeks receiving treatment for an inguinal hernia.

The parent bid me "good luck and a speedy recovery."

Her 12-year-old son, my orthodontic patient, overheard his mother's remark. He joined in expressing his good wishes with a "me too." This was quickly followed by, "But don't die! I don't want to wear these braces the rest of my life!" ❤

—Mitchell J. Burgin, DDS

My Young
Dental Assistant

n my experience, the key to success in working with children is the art of distraction. I show them all the equipment, starting with the suction tube, "Mr. Thirsty" for the younger set or the "Spit Sucker" for the more worldly. From there, I move on to the only magic trick I know—making water from a cup disappear before their very eyes with "Mr. Thirsty"—usually good to the last drop!

Once I get their undivided attention—providing I can persuade mom or dad to wait in the reception area, we move on to the "Magic Toothbrush" and the "Tooth Vitamins." I try and have kids sing with me as I count their teeth, checking for wobbly ones that could soon provide them with some income. That way, I'm quite successful in diverting their attention from the service I am trying to provide. If they're good, I reward them at the end of the treatment with a balloon animal (Should I quit dental hygiene and join the circus?), a new toothbrush, and finally a trip to the prize box. Usually, a good time is had by all with the bonus of returning in six months for yet more fun.

This one day, a young boy named Bryan sat in my chair for the first time. He seemed quite serious and in no mood for dental humor. Alas, my work was cut out for me. After a "ride" up and down in the dental chair and a full explanation of all my "cool tools," we were ready to begin.

As he didn't seem to be amused in the least, I decided distraction was called for. I had him hold a mirror with his left hand to watch and make sure I didn't forget any teeth. I also slipped the ring holding polishing paste onto the index finger of that same hand. And as if that wasn't enough, I asked him to hold the suction tube in his right hand. I made it seem that unless I enlisted his aid, we'd never get the job done. As I loaded him up with more and more tasks, I asked, "You don't expect me do *all* the work, do you?"

A look of concern crossed Bryan's face. Quite seriously and matter-of-factly he said, "You know, ma'am, my parents are *paying* you to do this...." I was speechless! ♥

—Judee Limardi, RDH

Fashion Statement

*I base most of my fashion taste
on what doesn't itch.*

—Gilda Radner

s pediatric specialists providing dental care for babies through teens, our work can be very physical. We kneel down to talk with toddlers, bend over to examine warm little wigglers, and dash to take those uncomfortable X rays as quickly as possible. Accordingly, the entire staff in our practice dresses quite practically in hospital "scrubs"—loose-fitting tunics and trousers featuring bright, seasonable colors of blue, yellow, pink, and olive. On our feet, we wear washable white sneakers. The outfits are always clean and comfortable.

One evening, dressed as a "civilian" in my finest gown for a gala benefit at the local hospital, I stopped at the grocery store. (I had to pick up an over-the-counter pain reliever for my son since we were running low at home. I knew before the night was over he would need relief from the discomfort of an orthodontic adjustment he'd had earlier that day.)

The market was packed. I picked up my pills and surveyed the enormous checkout queues. Finding the "12-item" line, I settled in—but not before several little patients of mine had discovered me. Bored with standing by their parents, they came over to confer with their dentist.

As this group consultation got under way, a bright-eyed, snaggle-toothed two-footer looked up and yelled exuberantly— for all the checkout lines to hear—"DR. MADIGAN, I DIDN'T RECOGNIZE YOU WITH YOUR CLOTHES ON!" ♥

—Ann Madigan, DMD, MSc

8

TOOTH FAIRY STORIES

Dear Tooth Fairy,
please do not take my tooth yet.
I have to show it
to my friends at school.

—Note left under pillow
(in place of tooth) by
Caroline Johnson, six years old
Submitted by her father,
Gregory R. Johnson, DDS

The Tooth Fairy

Just what does the Tooth Fairy do
After collecting teeth from me and you?
House to house, she gathers teeth in the night.
Astride a winged horse she takes her flight.

She flies through Great Britain and through Spain.
She flies through snow and sleet and rain.
Then on to Canada and the U.S. of A.
The Tooth Fairy works both night and day.

She needs thousands and thousands of teeth you see.
That's why she counts on you and me,
To shed our teeth so pearly white,
To place under pillows in the night.

If you awake and your tooth is still there,
Just relax, have no fear.
Plump up your pillow and pat it down tight,
The Tooth Fairy will come the following night.

Then she'll return to her castle, in the clouds, in the sky
She'll wash each tooth and gently pat it dry.
Carefully she'll sift the good from the bad.
Taking inventory, marking in her pad.

All the teeth that pass inspection will build her castle walls.
She'll build pillars and pathways, stairways and halls.
She'll make moats and bridges and wishing wells,
Trinkets, vases, and beautiful bells.

She weaves necklaces, watches, bracelets, and rings.
She makes wonderful, beautiful, fantastical things.
But the task from which she gets the most pride
Is sorting the "best teeth" and setting them aside.

These prize teeth get special billing,
They're not chipped or cracked or filled with filling.
The angels collect them and store them away
To brighten a baby's smile someday!

So keep your teeth strong with fluoride rinses
And they'll reside in a castle like a prince or a princess!
Or they may be in the next little baby's smile.
I couldn't think of anything more worthwhile! ♥

—Nancy Roe-Pimm, RDH

Notes from the Tooth Fairy

When we recall the past,
we find it is the simplest things—
not the great occasions—
that in retrospect give off
the greatest glow of happiness.

—Bob Hope

hen my two sisters and I were very young, our household filled with excitement whenever one of us had a loose tooth. We always waited impatiently for the tooth to finally relinquish its hold. That evening, the lucky girl placed her prized package ever so gently under her pillow. The next morning, we'd huddle around and examine the wonderfully witty, sometimes crazy, and always unique note from our "T.F.," as our Tooth Fairy called herself.

As we got older, we figured out just who the T.F. really was, as most kids do. Ours was our daddy. Actually, he was Gilbert S. Berman, DDS. Once in a while, our T.F. even had to help out a stubborn loose tooth before he went feverishly to work on the note for that evening.

Daddy's beloved T.F. notes were always creative and amusing. One was written backwards and could be read only in a mirror; another had been skillfully cut so that the recipient had to put the puzzle pieces together before the note could be read. There was one that had to be sung to the tune of "I've Been Workin' on the Railroad," and yet another that had been written in a spiral that made us dizzy to read. Another bonus of the T.F.'s communications was that "she" would always draw a picture of herself and add her signature.

Years later, I became a dental hygienist, got married, and had two great kids. When my oldest was six and her first tooth became loose, I knew I would continue the Tooth Fairy tradition. The thrill and pleasure of watching my kids read their T.F. notes—it seems I've inherited some of my dad's creativity—is very rewarding. I am certain the experience of losing their teeth and their relationship with their Tooth Fairy are memories my children will always cherish. I know mine are. Thanks, Daddy. ♥

—Shari Caplan, RDH

Mom, Are You Listening?

t was mid-December when a young patient came into our office and complained about a loose upper front tooth. To demonstrate its precarious condition, she wiggled it for us with her tongue.

The dentist asked if she wanted the tooth taken out.

The girl responded with an enthusiastic "Yesss!"

Without hesitation, the dentist snatched the tooth from her mouth with his already-gloved fingers before the child realized what was happening.

As the attending dental assistant, I asked the girl if she was going to place the tooth under her pillow for the Tooth Fairy.

"Yes," she replied, "but not tonight."

"Well then, just when *are* you planning to put the tooth under your pillow?"

"On Christmas Eve, silly, so the Tooth Fairy can meet Santa Claus." ❤

—Cathy Milejczak, CDA, RDH, BHS

Expensive Precedent

hen I asked Tommy how he was doing, the six-year-old informed me he had just lost a tooth. To back up his statement, he smiled really big, showing me the newly acquired gap in his dentition. I asked if the Tooth Fairy had made a visit.

"Yes!" Tommy said. "She gave me *20 dollars!*" His mother, standing next to him, proudly straightened herself while her face launched a knowing grin.

"Wow, Tommy! Did you know you have 19 more teeth to lose? You're going to be *rich!*"

Tommy's mother's grin started to fade, "Did you say *19* more?"

"Yes, 19 more teeth to lose!"

The stunned look that replaced the grin on her face was priceless. ❤

—Cheryl Lee Willett, DDS, MS

A Grain of Tooth

t's an exciting event when a child pulls out a loose tooth and places it carefully beneath his pillow at bedtime in the hope of finding it replaced the next morning with a dollar bill from the Tooth Fairy. On occasion, this simple process can pose a great challenge—both for the child and the Tooth Fairy.

Zach wiggled and pulled and twisted and pushed until, at last, his first baby tooth came out with a snap. Of course, his mouth started to bleed, and he frantically searched all his pockets until he found a wad of tissue to stanch the flow! Holding his tiny tooth in one hand and his mouth with the other, he scurried across the driveway toward the house.

Being a kid, he dropped his tooth along the way. Just as he stooped to pick it up, a chicken appeared out of nowhere and, mistaking the tooth for a piece of grain, picked it up in her beak. Now this particular chicken was not altogether stupid. Once she had the tooth, she realized it might not be edible and set it down to inspect it. Zach reached for the tooth again, but the hen was too fast. She seized his tooth and ran. Never one to give up easily, Zach took off after the hen as she zigzagged about. This attracted the attention of the rest of the chickens.

Again, the first hen set down her prize to examine it further. In an instant, the tooth was stolen by a second hen. The race was on, with Zach and the entire flock chasing the hen with the tooth.

Then the second hen set down the tooth to examine it—a foolish thing to do. Almost immediately, the tooth disappeared down the gullet of a third, less discriminating, bird. Poor Zach! Now what to do? How could the Tooth Fairy possibly make the exchange?

As he fed the chickens the following morning, Zach noticed that one hen was having a little trouble walking. Upon closer inspection, he observed a rolled-up dollar bill attached to her leg with a rubber band. At once, the chase took up where it left off the previous day! ❤

—Diane Brucato-Thomas, RDH, EF, BS

9

LEARNING FROM OUR PATIENTS

A moment's insight is sometimes worth a lifetime's experience.

—Oliver Wendell Holmes

Sam Eagle

To face despair and not give in to it.
That's courage.

—Ted Koppel

y friend died in October. I thought of him always, gone far too early, leaving me far too lonely. I was left with a packet of letters and pictures and the tape of Fogelberg songs that he'd recorded for me.

My staff and patients didn't know someone close to me had died; at least I didn't think so. I worked hard at maintaining quality and professionalism at work. But when I left work each night, I let the sadness overwhelm me. On the drive home, I'd slip the Fogelberg tape into the player and let it skewer my gut, never considering that forgoing it was a possibility, or that it was a *reminder* of the pain, not a remedy for it.

I kept my grief with me all through the early winter, shivering past December, through January, and on into Monday, the tenth of February. My assistant, Meg, met me in the hallway. "Sam Eagle's in the chair. Another abscess, he says." He'd had enough of them that I respected his self-diagnosis. I went to the treatment room and stopped to wash at the sink. The patient's chair faces the window, away from the door.

"Hello, Doc," he said, adjusting his bib. I smiled at his familiarity. "How's the Doc today?"

"Another abscess?" I asked.

"Yeah. Saturday night. Thanks for calling in the prescription." He twisted in the chair to see me. "The pharmacist knows me now." He grinned the grin that had cost him so much. Childhood care would have made such a difference for Sam.

Meg gave me the X-ray film she had just developed and a knowing look. Sam saw it. "Bad, huh?"

I pushed the film under the edging of the viewbox. "You've been on the Erythromycin since Saturday? Number of doses since then?" I asked.

"Six."

"We could open it today, get started," I suggested. Meg stood poised to gather the needed equipment.

"Okay, Doc."

"Go ahead, Meg. I'll get started here," I said.

I placed a swab of topical anesthetic by Sam's premolar. His fingertips rested on his bib. His nails were broad and scarred with his history of injuries. He'd been in casts and bandages many times through the years I'd known him. He'd begun telling me each visit how he wanted to get out of mechanics, but nothing offered dental benefits, he'd laugh, or paid as well.

"How's the job search going?" I asked.

He looked down his nose at his bib. "Ah, bad. Lousy bad. Nothing yet. I might even get discouraged."

That was it. That was all it took. Any bit of reverie or regret brought my sadness right to the forefront. For four months I'd felt like a gaping wound.

I slipped an anesthetic cartridge into the syringe and slid the shaft into place. I shimmied the cap from the needle and encircled Sam's head in my arm. He tipped his face, knowing just the position I needed. I placed the syringe and gently pulled his lip over the tip. He sighed and his fingers flattened onto the bib. Then, seduced by the comfort of his familiarity, I did something stupid. "I'm in a rut, too," I said—instantly regretting it.

Sam's eyes popped wide, a furrow creased his brow, and I felt him tense. As eager to chat as a patient may be, they don't want to hear that their dentist is depressed. I attempted quick repairs. "Winter, you know. Back and forth, Vineland to Cape May to Vineland to Cape May. Throw in Stone Harbor for errands. That rut. Winter just blocks me in...so dark at night." I babbled, growing the lie, making it worse. At that point, I just wanted to be driving home.

Finally the cartridge was empty. I retracted the syringe and rolled my chair away from Sam's, out of that intimate zone we dentists invade, but that day it was *I* who needed the personal space.

I felt Sam's eyes upon me as I capped the syringe. I knew he was waiting for eye contact.

"You know what another name for a rut is, don't you Doc?"

"No, what's that?"

"A grave, only longer."

Meg came in with the rubber dam tray, and I placed the clamp on Sam's premolar. His back arched, then relaxed, and I read in his eyes that he relented for now. I began the root canal, accessing and shaping the chamber, then positioning a film for the X ray.

Waiting for the film to develop, I slumped into my misery, just as I did each day when I listened to that tape on the drive home. My sadness had become a habit by then, as pacifying as a favorite sweatshirt. Slipping into it was so soothing. I indulged it selfishly and didn't regard its eclipse of all around me.

Meg handed me the film. "We have our working length. That's as far as I'll go today. Next time we'll shape and seal." I medicated and temporized. Sam watched the reflection in my glasses as I eased the clamp from his tooth. Meg checked his bite as I gave homecare instructions.

I moistened a gauze square and concentrated on dabbing at some temporary cement on Sam's cheek. It was a job requiring no concentration at all, but I needed to delay the questions I felt certain he'd ask me. I knew his eyes were on mine, patiently waiting.

"Done?" he asked.

"Yes." I looked at him then, at such close range as we were, and braced for the questions. But it wasn't questions he gave me. He lifted his hand from his bib and placed it on mine. For all its coarse appearance, the touch was gentle.

He spoke softly, "If you put a ramp at the end of that rut, it's not a grave anymore." His eyes held me tight.

The operatory, the chair, everything about us, blurred, and I saw only his eyes. And in them I saw that there was indeed an alternative to the despair that I'd nurtured all those months. I saw there was a course of hope and acceptance, and of grander things. And I saw that the compassion of a patient could illuminate them, and I opened my heart to them.

That night I drove home in silence, the Fogelberg tape on the seat, with Sam's words helping me steer. ♥

—Helen Jasnosz, DDS

Life Lessons

Be kind—everyone you meet is fighting a hard battle.

—Plato

s I drove to work at Dr. Sherman's dental office, I turned off the car radio and used the time to take inventory of my life. My husband and I have built a fine marriage during our 12 years together, we have four healthy children, and I have a wonderful part-time job as a dental hygienist. (What a great profession for a woman who's raising a family!) The flexibility allows me to stay active in the profession without feeling the time with my children is being compromised. A friend and neighbor baby-sits for me one day a week. She has children close in age to my own, and they enjoy being together. I also work Saturdays, allowing my husband real quality time with our children.

Smugly I thought to myself, *I am the epitome of a modern-day woman...juggling a job and family and somehow making it all work!* After that mental pat on the back, I thought about the day ahead. I enjoyed chatting with people and found cleaning their teeth somewhat therapeutic—for *me* as well as for my patients! Patients came in needing a service, and in the course of an hour, I would evaluate their dental health, teach them effective oral hygiene techniques, and send each one off with a clean and fresh-feeling mouth! I really loved my job. Having a day and a half a week to work outside the home provided an additional benefit—a stimulating change of pace, *the opportunity to talk to people over nine years old.*

The afternoon began quite typically. After my first patient, I cleaned and bagged the instruments and disinfected the operatory. I placed a new toothbrush and floss on the tray next to a new set of instruments and poured some minty mouth rinse into a cup.

Reviewing the chart of the next patient, I realized Mrs. Douglas was someone I'd never met. It had been almost two years since her previous teeth cleaning. *Uh oh!* I thought. *I'll have to remind her of the importance of regular dental visits.*

As I called Mrs. Douglas from the waiting room, I noticed that her thinning black hair was streaked with gray. Her face was oval shaped and accented with dark brown eyes. Her olive skin was makeup-free and marked with deep lines around her eyes and mouth. She had a hard look about her. I was taken aback by her unpleasant facial expression and avoidance of eye contact. *What's her problem?* I wondered. *I'm only running about five minutes behind!* Patients that came in with an attitude really irritated me. *Whatever made your day so miserable wasn't my fault,* I thought to myself.

"You may have a seat in Room One, Mrs. Douglas. May I take your coat?" I asked gently, trying to soften her up.

"*No!* I'll keep it with me," she snapped.

Looking at her health history, I asked if there were any changes in her health since her last visit.

"*No!*" was her curt response. I thought this might be the appropriate time to comment on the need for six-month dental cleanings as opposed to two years! In a tactful way, I had to let her know she had been very lax in caring for her teeth.

As I mentioned the importance of regular six-month checkups to insure healthy teeth and gums, Mrs. Douglas looked at me as if I had no idea what I was talking about.

She took a deep breath, peered at my face through her watery brown eyes, and explained why she had been so overdue for her dental appointment. She said her husband, Rob, had spent the last year and a half battling colon cancer. He had endured major surgery and a long course of radiation. Just one and a half years ago, he had been an active 63-year-old whose disease was discovered at his annual physical. His life, and the life of his family, spiraled out of control from that day on. Mrs. Douglas was there for him through it all; recovery from the surgery, special diets, medication, discomforts, and sickness caused by a rigorous course of radiation.

Despite his determination and the efforts of his physicians, Mr. Douglas lost his battle with cancer three months earlier. Mrs. Douglas couldn't help but smile as she told me what a wonderful man Rob had been. It was obvious how much she missed her life's partner. Loneliness was her regular companion now. With misty eyes, she looked at me and said, "You never know when your life can be turned upside down in an instant. Don't ever take your loved ones for granted." As we continued with her appointment, my whole demeanor changed. It was heartwarming and humbling to see my patient's emotional relief in talking through her feelings and experiences.

n the way home from work that night, I offered a prayer for Mrs. Douglas. She had touched me by sharing the challenges of her husband's journey down cancer's rocky road. I had had the opportunity to truly connect with Mrs. Douglas and share her pain. I couldn't help but feel pangs of guilt, thinking about how I had initially judged her. I once again reminded myself that our patients are whole human beings. We really don't know what experiences, joys, and sadness they bring with them when they sit down in our dental chair. It is a privilege to have the chance to reach out to other people one on one. As a dental hygienist, I sometimes have the honor of sharing my knowledge about periodontal disease and effective hygiene techniques. However, more often than you might think, it is I who learn valuable life lessons from my patients. ❤

—Kathleen E. Banas, RDH

Little Billy

*The common denominator of all healing methods
is unconditional love—a love that respects
the uniqueness of each individual.*

—Jack Schwartz

y first employment as a young dentist fresh out of school was in a community public health clinic in West Seattle. I didn't think it would turn into a long-term commitment, but I vowed I would spend two years there to gain speed and experience and then transfer into private practice. The clinic was located in the same neighborhood that I had been born into 27 years earlier. The nostalgia of being back there felt good to me. It was almost as if I had been called back for some reason.

The clinic was set up to treat children from low-income families. Many of the children we saw were from broken homes, dysfunctional families, and abusive environments. It didn't take long to realize that there were many more things to learn about people and teeth that were not included in the dental school curriculum. I had learned what to do, but now I was going to learn how to do it. Unique experiences and learning opportunities presented themselves almost every day.

One of my earliest experiences was when little six-year-old Billy came in for his first dental checkup. He had a mouth full of cavities and other dental problems that would require numerous appointments in order to treat them properly. I could tell he was nervous and that he seemed unusually wary of the whole experience. I wondered how he would do for the actual dental procedures and if I had the necessary management skills to complete the extensive treatment plan and still provide a positive experience for both him and me.

When he returned for his next appointment the answer came quickly. He totally freaked out! We had barely even started when he began crying and yelling and thrashing about. He was frantic—filled with irrational fear. He kicked and hit and spit and bit, shredded his bib and his chart, and tried breaking the dental equipment, scattering the instruments across the floor. He was like a caged animal, totally panic-stricken and out of control!

The management techniques I learned in school to deal with this kind of behavior consisted of physically restraining the patient, firmly but gently, so that he couldn't hurt himself. At the same time you held one hand over his mouth to stifle his yells and to limit the amount of oxygen that was available to him. This promised to get his attention so that you could look directly into the patient's eyes and instruct him to calm down. You were not supposed to remove your hand from his mouth until he complied with your request. It all sounded good when I learned about it, but in practice it didn't work for little Billy or me. In his state of mind, he was way stronger than I was, and it was a no-holds-barred survival match as far as he was concerned. I held on as long as I could, but it only seemed to increase his conviction to escape. His flailing frenzy and irrational hysteria grew in intensity. It was difficult under these circumstances to convince him that I was trying to help him and meant him no harm. I finally gave up. Afterward, I felt exhausted and traumatized and was sure that he felt the same way, too.

His deteriorated dental condition needed help, and I knew that I was his only resource. Deep down inside I knew there must be a better way to win him over. I prayed for guidance and mentally searched for the solution. I decided to forget about doing dentistry on him for a while and just be his friend. I scheduled him to come back and took him to the small community park across the street from the duplex that we were using as the clinic.

He was tense and resistant at first, but as I pushed him on the swings and helped him down the slide he started to have fun. I hoisted him up on my shoulders and ran around, bouncing him up and down, back and forth across the park and down an adjoining alley. He was having the time of his life, laughing and yelling at the top of his lungs, and I was feeling enthused that this approach seemed to be working. We returned to the swings, and as I was pushing him again, a police car pulled up to the curb and two of the biggest cops I had ever seen got out and started walking in our general direction.

Little Billy seemed very excited to see them and started screeching, *"Police! Police!"*

I assumed there was a local domestic disturbance going on nearby and they were here to check it out. But, they came right over to us and started asking me questions. They wanted to know who I was, what I was doing, what kind of car I drove, and where it was. I explained who I was and what I was doing and why, and that my wife had dropped me off at work so that she could use our black sedan for the day.

They didn't buy my story. Without saying why or checking at the clinic, they said they would have to take me down to the police station for more questioning. I was scared and couldn't believe this was happening! There was no convincing them any differently. Just as I was being assisted into the patrol car, the clinic's hygienist, who knew I was at the park, nonchalantly walked out with some X rays for me to look at. She was totally surprised by the police action and quickly identified me as the dentist, verifying that I was trying to help little Billy get over his fears of needed dental work.

The police then explained that there was a child abuser loose in the area and that a neighbor had called them when she heard Billy's yelling. I just happened to match the villain's description; and the type of car he was seen in was a dark-colored sedan.

The police apologized and praised me for what I was doing. Then the bigger and taller one leaned over, pulled little Billy right up close, into his face, and said to him, "You listen to this dentist and do what he says or you'll end up like this!" He suddenly spit out his two partial dentures, dangling them from the front edge of his lips!

The sight of those artificial teeth ejecting out of his mouth totally shocked me; poor little Billy's eyes got bigger than baseballs. He must have been thoroughly jolted and perplexed by the unnerving spectacle.

 don't know if little Billy ever realized what had actually happened, but after we both recovered from the disturbing display, we walked hand in hand back to the clinic. I knew I had made a new friend, and little Billy was a model patient ever since that day.

I don't know if it was the cop, me, or the combination of both that made the difference, but I knew my prayer for guidance had been answered. I discovered that the underlying common ground that everyone responded to was Love. I learned that children are especially sensitive to Love's vibration. The primary method of communication for children is more nonverbal than verbal. The younger they are, the more they rely on physical cues for information about their world. They respond to the quality of your touch, the vibration of the sounds and motions you make, and the intention registered in your gaze. Their ability to accurately communicate through feelings is developed long before their capacity for understanding spoken language.

It took me several years to perfect this management technique. It requires consciously creating an atmosphere that is filled with the good intentions of helping and loving others. You learn to fill the room with your countenance of joy, nurturing, honor, and respect, producing a climate of genuine caring. It is communicated through your touch, your voice, your posture, and your look. When you look at someone, you purposely look past their physical form and interact with the Divine essence of Life that dwells inside each body that unites us all into Oneness. This acknowledgment of their greatness is felt by the patient, and they respond with trust.

Thank you for teaching me this invaluable lesson, little Billy. ♥

—Sherwin R. Shinn, DDS

Punctured Ego

I hated the dentist I went to as a child, although I found out much later that he was a well-respected pedodontist—children's specialist. Why I decided to become a dentist, in spite of this, is another story.

When I was a dental student, I decided that I never wanted a child to feel about me the way I felt about my first dentist. After setting up my practice, I was especially concerned about the need to give my young patients a dreaded "shot" before preparing their teeth for fillings. I had learned many little tricks in dental school to help make this situation as uneventful as possible.

One day I had a seven-year-old girl come in for her first filling and tried extra hard to be as gentle and clever as I could so as not to upset her. I had a glass syringe that was smaller and lighter than the typical metal ones—I could practically palm it. I told her I was going to squirt a little "sleepy juice" around her tooth and applied some topical anesthetic to the area. I tipped the operating light up just enough to get in her eyes a bit and had my assistant pass me the syringe under her chin—just as I had been taught—so that the child couldn't see it. As I started to inject the anesthetic, I jiggled her lip and cheek as a distraction—just as I had been taught. Success! Through the whole injection—which I did very slowly, just as I had been taught—she didn't bat an eyelash.

The rest of the appointment was uneventful. I was feeling

rather proud of my technique and wanted to let Mom know how good I was—in a subtle way, of course.

Before I could get to the reception room, however, the young lady jumped out of the dental chair, swerved around me, and raced to her mother. Then, in a voice loud enough for all to hear, she announced: *"Mommie, Mommie! The dentist gave me a shot, and he doesn't even think I know it!"* ❤

—Robert E. Lavine, DDS

Dental Détente

ast year I had the opportunity to welcome a new family into my practice. George, an American, had married and brought to this country a woman from the Ukraine. Sasha and her teenage sons, Boris and Yuri, were a delight. They dressed neatly, spoke fine English, and were getting used to American life—including fast food! Sasha, who grew up in the days of the old Soviet Union, was constantly in awe of our supermarkets, shopping malls, and freeways.

Unfortunately, all three of these patients needed a lot of dental treatment. There were broken fillings, half-filled root canals, abscessed teeth, large cavities, and old gold bridges and crowns in sad disrepair. Their oral hygiene also had to improve. They had seen dentists in the Ukraine, so it was obvious Sasha cared about their dental health. But unfortunately, all the old work had to be redone.

My challenge was to present the treatment plan without downgrading the previous work or embarrassing my new patients. With her new husband at her side, the mother questioned me, repeatedly asking, "Why is it you need to do *this*?" Her concern was understandable. I knew Sasha just wanted to make sure that she and her sons got the best.

George's new family knew little about proper flossing or brushing, and even less about the effect of diet on teeth and gums. One by one, I described the simple techniques they could initiate at home—consistent steps to improve their dental health. I believed my positive approach would delight both dedicated parents. But every patient has a unique perspective—a view all their own. Finally, Sasha asked me to compare the state of dentistry in our two countries.

As I reviewed the exceptional dental technologies available in America, my patient took a mental side trip—back to the Ukraine. With somber eyes she looked up at me and managed one simple defense of her homeland: "Our *rockets* are better, no?"

Rockets? I did a quick mental detour of my own and burst into laughter.

"Yes, Sasha!" I answered. "*Absolutely!* You come from the land of great cosmonauts. I will make sure the dental treatment we provide for you and your sons will be every bit as good as your rockets." With that reassurance, she smiled and consented to the proposed treatment plan. ♥

—Richard L. Plasch, DDS, FAGD

A Bad Day

Just think how happy you'd be if you lost everything and everyone you have right now, and then, somehow got everything back again.

—Kobi Yamada

thought the day would never end. Only a couple of weeks remained until Christmas, and I felt overwhelmed with so much still to be done. My three boys all needed something, grandma and mother-in-law expected me to do their shopping, there were cookies to bake, a tree to trim, and lots of shopping of my own to finish. Fortunately, the last patient scheduled for that afternoon was a very pleasant elderly lady I had met six months earlier. I knew the hour would go by quickly.

Eighty-five years young, Mrs. Carwile greeted me with a bright smile and a friendly hello. After her cleaning, we waited for the doctor to come in and perform his exam. Simply to make conversation, I asked Mrs. Carwile about her holiday plans and how her family was.

She replied, "No, Mary, I have no family...except for my church family, that is."

"You never got married or had children?" I asked.

Mrs. Carwile stared out the window for a moment as if in a daydream before responding. Softly and calmly, she said, "Oh yes, dear, I had all of that. But about 50 years ago, my husband

and two baby girls, ages three and four, were killed in a car accident. I survived. I decided that my loss was far too great to ever start over, so I chose to be content alone with my fond memories of them."

Suddenly, my bad day didn't seem so bad after all. As the Christmas holidays drew nearer and I bought gifts for my sons, did the shopping for grandma and mother-in-law, baked cookies, trimmed the tree, and finished my own shopping, I constantly reminded myself just how fortunate I was to have a family to care for. ❤

—Mary Cole, RDH

He Cared

Life's most persistent and urgent question is:
What are you doing for others?

—Dr. Martin Luther King, Jr.

s the New Year rolled in, it gave me pause to look over the latest calendar. I noticed that the first holiday after New Year was to be Martin Luther King, Jr. Day. Our newest holiday, it always made me a little envious of today's children who have the day off from school. I think to myself, "What I could have done with that day off when I was nine."

I'll be at work on Martin Luther King, Jr. Day. And like many other holidays, I'll get to visit with the children who have the day off from school and whose parents know this is a great time to bring little Johnny to the dentist. And like many other holidays, I will inquire of my young friends, "Why do you have today off from school?"

Once I was curious to know if my youngsters knew who Dr. Martin Luther King was and why his birthday was a holiday. I asked one little boy of about eight, and he couldn't come up with an answer. He had no idea; and the response he did give was not pleasant. I began to wonder if schools were overlooking the importance of Dr. King's contributions to our society. Undaunted, I continued to survey my young patients.

In the early afternoon, a little girl visited our office. During the course of her examination, I asked why she didn't have school that day.

To my surprise, she quickly responded, "Martin Luther King."

Wondering what she knew about Dr. King, I continued by asking, "What did he do?" There was a pause...she was thinking. I too was thinking. I was thinking what a tragedy that all these children have the day off from school and don't know why. I coaxed her a little more, "Come on, what did he do? You know."

The first-grader looked me in the eye, and in a small but sure voice, answered, "He cared."

Her words echoed in my mind. *"He cared."*

I learned something that day...something about myself and about a special little girl. Since then, Dr. King's birthday has never been the same for me. That child brought tears to my eyes. In all her innocence, she knew what counted. I had tears because someday, like most of us, she'll probably forget what counts. I had tears because maybe I wasn't talking to a little first-grader at all. Maybe for that one brief, tiny moment, God was talking to me. Six years later I still can't forget it. ❤

—John R. Grasso, DDS

10

THANK YOU, THANK YOU!

*Gratitude unlocks the fullness of life. It
turns what we have
into enough and more.*

—Melody Beattie

Oh, I Have a Terrible Pain in My Head!

*One of the most sublime experiences we can have
is to wake up feeling healthy after we have been sick.
Even if it is only relief from a headache or toothache,
the health we take for granted most of the time
is suddenly seen to be an incredible blessing.*

—Harold Kushner

he plane engines droned their purposeful sounds while I was cocooned in the privacy of my window seat reading the latest "best book" en route from our Phoenix home to a speaking engagement in Miami, Florida.

"As we prepare for landing, please check to see that your seat belt is securely fastened, your seat back and tray table are in their full upright and locked position, and all carry-on baggage is safely stowed under the seat in front of you or in the overhead compartment," the public address system commanded.

I reluctantly closed my book, raised my head, and looked out the window while adjusting to the reality of our Miami arrival. And then it happened! I felt something I had never felt before and exclaimed to my husband, Jim, "Oh, I have a terrible pain in my head!"

At the same time, the thought flashed through my mind, "I've never, ever, reached for a painkiller—not even a simple aspirin—for a mere 'headache.' " But what I was feeling at that moment was a totally new kind of pain—pain the likes of which I had never experienced before.

Jim and I had been speaking professionally for years, mostly in the healthcare field and primarily to the dental profession. Sitting there on the plane with the throbbing in my head, I asked myself how I could possibly manage to speak for two hours the next morning—and another two hours the following afternoon.

Thus began a six-month nightmare that only those who have experienced continual, excruciating pain can identify with. Thus also began the journey to find the cause of my agony! The healthcare professionals I consulted during the next six months included a family practitioner, a neurologist, a pain control/biofeedback specialist, and a massage/acupressure therapist—all to no avail! Of course, throughout this ordeal, there was always lots and lots of prayer!

As the months passed, each healthcare specialty did its very best with tests, CAT scans, medications, questions, counseling, and encouragement. However, no cause seemed to surface. It wasn't long before I began a downward emotional spiral as I tried to cope with the awesome reality of intense lifelong pain. I seriously began to wonder how long my tolerance would allow me to even function for short intervals—on the speaking platform and in the other areas of my life.

Several months later, when Jim and I were speaking at a dental conference in Vancouver, Canada, our host dentist asked if I had ever been challenged with TMJ pain. I said that I had, so he made me a bite splint in the hope that this would relieve my suffering.

From Vancouver, our next speaking engagement took us to

Dallas, Texas. By this time, my routine had become set. Breakfast in the room, dress, speak, go back to bed until the afternoon, dress, speak, and return to bed until the next flight.

We were picked up at the Dallas airport by our host, Dr. Bill White. We apologetically explained my "routine" and declined an invitation to a lovely dinner so that I could rest in preparation for fulfilling the privileged obligation of our next day's session.

Because the bite splint seemed to need some adjusting, Dr. White suggested I meet him at his office the next morning before the start of the day's conference activity. I arrived with all the resolve—and "make-up"—needed to endure the opening session.

As he seated me in the dental chair, Dr. White asked, "What happened to you just before the headache started?"

Oh, I thought to myself, that question has been asked by every practitioner I had seen in the previous six months! In exasperation, I replied, "Nothing happened TO ME!" This response was followed by a long pause as Dr. White considered my words.

"Naomi, what happened to someone else?" Breakthrough! Oh, the power of a person, a professional, a health professional, who chooses to REALLY LISTEN! This dentist "heard" what I did not realize I had said!

"Oh, nothing really. Well...EXCEPT...my dear friend, Bonnie, broke her leg crossing a creek in northern Arizona," I murmured.

"What did that have to do with you?" he asked.

"I was with her at the time and, in the hour-long drive to the hospital in Flagstaff, I knelt in the back of their Jeep Wagoneer and applied pressure between her foot and her knee. If I relaxed the pressure, even the slightest, she would scream in pain. But that was a full two weeks before my headache started!"

There was another long pause before Dr. White said, "Naomi, there are two muscles in your shoulders that are hard as a rock. I'm going to push on them and hold the pressure for ten seconds. The procedure will be extremely painful, but I will release after just ten seconds."

For each of those ten seconds the pain was so intense I thought I would die. But then...but then...but then...I had NO PAIN in my head! It was almost a FULL MINUTE before the pain returned. But what had changed totally for me was that HOPE had entered my reality.

nly in Dr. White's office did I finally realize that my concern for Bonnie and her pain had superseded the need to release the muscle tension in my own shoulders during that hour-long ride to the Flagstaff hospital. Two weeks after that incident, the positioning of my head for the long hours of reading on the flight from Phoenix to Miami became the "second accident," and the mystery pain was the result.

After many months of ultrasonic therapy, massage therapy, and chiropractic treatment—all on the muscles in my shoulders and back—I once again enjoyed the comfort of a pain-free head. I was able once again to look forward to a speaking schedule that could be accomplished with joy. And my heart was overflowing with praise to God for a dentist who listened not only for what *was* said, but for what *was not* said! A dentist who went far beyond what was expected, far beyond the physiology of dental pain. A dentist who cared about the person—the patient—as *a whole being!*

He became a true hero to me—the facilitator of a healthy, purpose-filled life, a professional *par excellence*. Thank you, Dr. White. Thank you, thank you, thank you! ♥

—Naomi Rhode, RDH, CSP
CPAE Speaker Hall of Fame

No Charge, Professor

The only people with whom you should try to get even are those who have helped you.

—Mae Maloo

ome time ago, the Georgetown University Dental School in Washington, D.C. established a new Department of Community Dentistry and I was asked to serve as its chair. Our department provided lectures and other activities for all classes, from freshman through senior. In the process, my colleagues and I had the opportunity to closely observe the progress of our students, and we got to know many of them—as well as their qualifications— rather well.

At age 65, I retired. Ten years later as a white-haired, arthritic old professor, I broke a tooth. On those rare occasions when I needed a little dentistry, I had relied on the services of a fellow faculty member in Washington. However my broken tooth was a major problem requiring immediate attention, and at age 75, I wasn't eager to navigate the heavy traffic in our nation's capital. Instead, I decided to visit the office of Dr. Alan Hinkle in a Washington suburb near my home because I remembered that he had been an outstanding student.

As I expected, the fractured tooth proved unsalvageable. Following the extraction, Dr. Hinkle refused to accept any money. When my gum had healed, I returned to his office for impressions so that a permanent bridge could be produced to replace the lost tooth. Since the special type of bridge to be made was typically quite expensive, I told him I insisted on paying—at the very least—a reduced "professional courtesy" fee.

In due time, Dr. Hinkle made a fine bridge. After he had cemented it in, he accompanied me to the waiting room where I inquired of his receptionist what the fee was. "Nothing, Dr. Christopher—those are my orders."

I turned to Dr. Hinkle, "C'mon, Alan, you can at least let me pay the lab bill!"

Dr. Hinkle looked me in the eyes, smiled, put both hands on my shoulders, and said, "When I feel I'm giving you more than you gave me, then I'll start to charge you."

I was embarrassed and overwhelmed. I don't know what came over me, but I started to cry. The dentist and his receptionist asked if I was okay. "I'm alright," I answered as I wiped away the tears. "Your generosity went right to my heart—it really got to me." Moments later, glowing with the experience of receiving love and kindness from a very caring human being, this white-haired old teacher left for the parking lot. ❤

—Andrew Christopher, BS, DDS, MHA, FICD
(Retired)

Agnes and
Her Precious Gift

Joy comes not to him who seeks it for himself,
but to him who seeks it for other people.

—H.S. Sylvester

y wife, Sandy, a dental hygienist, and I were assigned to a mission hospital dental department in Kenya, East Africa. One morning at sick call, a small woman named Agnes reported to our clinic. She was extremely thin and looked "dry," as they say in Africa. Our new patient filled out the necessary forms and we were told she had had an accident almost a month earlier. We did our examination and took X rays. To our dismay, we discovered swelling inside and out on her face and mouth, several severely fractured teeth, multiple semi-healed lacerations within the mouth, and a fractured jaw that had already begun to form a callus at the fracture site.

When we started asking Agnes questions about her accident, she became very quiet; and then large tears formed in her eyes. We assured Agnes that while we didn't want to upset her, we were very concerned about what had caused the injuries. We indicated she was going to need a lot of care. With continuing tears, she told us she had no money to pay for treatment but that she was in so much pain she could no longer tolerate it.

All of us on the staff put our heads together and determined we could come up with enough from our own pockets to cover her treatment. When we told Agnes we would be able to provide care without cost to her, she stopped crying and almost smiled. We treated her conditions by removing the teeth that could not be saved and repairing the rest. We repositioned and sutured some of the lacerations and tissue flaps. Because her bite was not badly out of alignment, we elected not to reset her broken jaw.

Once Agnes's mouth was anesthetized, she began to smile, telling us that this was the first time in a month she had been without pain. As we proceeded with her care, she gained more confidence in us and appreciated our concern. She told us she had been beaten by her intoxicated husband and had been picked up bodily and tossed out of her home. Badly injured, she had traveled many miles to her parents' village and tolerated the pain because her family had no money to pay for treatment.

Learning about the clinic, Agnes had walked many hours through the forest to reach our facility. We arranged transportation home for her and asked that she return in one week so that we could check the healing and remove her sutures.

When Agnes came back, she was all smiles as she hugged each of us. She was a very different lady—no swelling, healing satisfactorily, and no pain. We removed the sutures and pronounced her well on the road to recovery. Smiling again, Agnes reached into her bag and handed us three fresh eggs, gave us hugs again, and said she was sorry that that was all that she could give us, but she knew God would bless us all.

Every one of us on the mission team agreed that He had, indeed, blessed us with gifts of far greater value than money—or scarce fresh eggs: Agnes's warm smiles and hugs. ❤

—Robert J. Harland, DMD

The Art of Appreciation

We make a living by what we get,
but we make a life by what we give.

—Winston Churchill

arly in my career I was frequently on call for emergencies. These weeklong periods presented numerous challenges and often necessitated last-minute changes in my office schedule and personal plans. Admittedly, I was prone to complaining about the chaos that often accompanied "being on call."

On one such occasion I was summoned to my office on a Sunday afternoon to see a young boy named Paul. I met a very frightened five-year-old and his parents at the front door. Paul was in obvious discomfort with visible facial swelling. A subsequent examination and X ray revealed an abscessed molar. Further investigation revealed numerous other areas of decay on all posterior teeth and lesions on each of the erupting six-year molars.

While I treated Paul, his parents told me they had recently immigrated to Canada from the Ukraine following the Chernobyl nuclear disaster. Mother and father were deeply concerned about the long-term effects the resulting radioactive fallout might have on their three children and left excellent university positions to seek a new life.

I proceeded that day to extract the offending tooth after

being able to obtain good anesthesia despite the swelling. Antibiotics were prescribed and I recommended that Paul return in 48 hours for a postoperative visit. As we left the operatory I realized that Paul's parents were noticeably concerned about how they were going to pay for the visit. Paul reminded me a lot of my own five-year-old son, Christopher, so I told them there would be no fee. After offering me profuse thanks, the family left the office.

The following week, Paul's father presented me with a beautiful landscape oil painting done by a talented family friend in Russia. This painting now graces my home and has served as a constant reminder throughout my career that, despite the inevitable ups and downs of our professional lives, we are truly blessed with the opportunity to serve others. This outshines any monetary gain we might seek and offers each of us far greater rewards.

Paul returned to the office many times during the first year of treatment. My partner and I were pleased to help him regain excellent oral health. His father was able to secure employment during that year, and the whole family remained patients of our office for more than a decade until they moved from our area.

The painting remains on my wall offering a constant reminder of the valuable lesson Paul's first visit taught me. Dentistry offers all of us a rare opportunity to make an impact on other people's lives. In the process, we can learn a lot about ourselves. ❤

—Ian W. Tester, DDS

Once Again, Thank You!

Bear ye one another's burdens.

—Galatians 6:2

n February 1, 1996, a major crisis burst into our lives: my wife, Nancy, was diagnosed with ovarian cancer. My dedicated staff joined in the efforts to help our family deal with the struggles that accompanied such horrible news. After she survived the emergency hysterectomy and the first three rounds of chemotherapy that followed, I decided it was time to treat Nancy to a mini-vacation.

Two days after we left on our trip, we were hit with another tragedy. My partner of 17 years, Dr. Kulik—the man with whom I had just built a new dental office—was involved in a hideous traffic accident. He required ten hours of emergency surgery to reattach his left arm that was practically torn off by a passing vehicle.

Nancy and I cut our trip short and returned to South Bend where she received her last three rounds of chemotherapy. We now had two practices in one facility with only one dentist whose wife was in a major health crisis. With the God-sent help of my staff, Dr. Kulik's staff, and more than 50 volunteers from the North Central Dental Society in South Bend filling in for Dr. Kulik, we somehow survived! For the last five years, we have operated "one day at a time!"

Following her last round of chemotherapy, Nancy spent

several weeks in Chicago where she received a bone marrow transplant. Back then, my staff got used to changing schedules, times, and procedures with little or no warning. They did anything they could to make our lives easier during this difficult period. They were—and continue to be—quite unbelievable in their love, support, and caring for my practice, my patients, and, above all, my family.

My partner, Dr. Kulik, has endured numerous surgeries since his accident and—four years later—continues to receive regular physical therapy. The good news is that he is now able to maintain a four-and-a-half-days-a-week work schedule. His staff has diligently maintained their support, caring, and help towards Dr. Kulik and his family during the most difficult time in *their* lives! And as long as I'm sharing good news, I'll pass along the fact that Nancy's cancer has responded well to her treatment—she has been in full remission since her bone marrow transplant in 1996!

Looking back, I realize it would have been impossible for me to endure these tragedies without occasionally looking for the lighter side. In those rare moments, I still kid our staffs about how they had a priest bless our office building when we opened the doors. I know the man used holy water, but I think he might have gotten his bottles mixed up!

egardless of the tough and trying times we two dentists, and our families, have had in recent years, we can count our blessings for the wonderful human beings we work with. They will be in our hearts forever. No words can thank them for what they have done. I am the luckiest man in the world to be privileged to work with each and every one of them. God bless them all; and once again, thank you! ❤

—Daniel E. White, DDS

A Thousand Hugs

Love received, and love given,
comprise the best form of therapy.

—Gordon Allport

 started my career as a dental hygienist working for a young dentist in a suburban neighborhood. The homes of many of our patients were just a short distance from the office. As a result, some of our grade school patients would walk to the office for their dental appointments. A few routinely stopped by just to say hello on their way home after school. Several of these children and I became friends, and I looked forward to seeing them often.

One morning as I got up to get ready for work, I became aware that my apartment was full of smoke. A few seconds later, I realized the entire building was engulfed in flames. Trying hard not to panic, I awakened my roommate, and we quickly prepared to escape. As I opened our apartment door, I immediately felt searing pain in my hands and on my face. The fire had made our metal apartment door so intensely hot that the skin on my hands was instantly burned. At the hospital, I was diagnosed with third-degree burns on both hands and second-degree burns on my face.

My roommate and I were put in separate isolation rooms to prevent infection. Only our immediate families were allowed to visit, and they had to be covered with protective clothing from head to toe. The isolation also meant we couldn't have any flowers, balloons, or get-well gifts.

When my patients heard what had happened and that I wouldn't be back for some time, the children became very upset because they couldn't see me or send get-well flowers. One of my coworkers came up with a solution that made both the patients and me feel better. She got crayons and paper, and the children designed get-well greetings for me while visiting the office. She then sealed the drawings in clear plastic bags, normally used for sterilizing instruments, and brought them to the nurse's station. Then, members of the hospital staff would tape the plastic bags to my isolation room walls.

Each time I received a delivery of drawings, I felt as if those children were giving me a thousand get-well hugs. After I recovered from the skin grafts, I returned to work anxious to once again see the children who had given me hope and to return their love-filled hugs in person. ♥

—Jackie S. Perry, RDH, BSDH

A Letter for My Father

t was a day before New Years. I was unpacking boxes in our very first house, a cottage for Ray, our little John, and me. We were urban appliqués on a patchwork of dairies: Rising Sun, Maryland, next to the Pennsylvania line. Also the Delaware line and the Mason-Dixon line—we were near to everywhere and close to nothing.

That afternoon, John was my household elf, a jester and minstrel at seven. He paraded about with a tambourine until I unpacked (*voilà!*) a medieval wooden flute. So began our short-lived revels. While I played, John twirled and pranced. And with a sudden courtly flourish, he planted the flute straight up into the roof of my mouth, driving a front tooth into Shakespearean realms of pain and gore. I screamed, I bled, I disinherited my son. He fled to the asylum well known to small assailants: the underworld beneath his bed.

Eventually, I had the presence of mind to free and pardon my child. There was a more pressing issue to deal with, and it wasn't under John's bed. It was one-sixteenth of an inch deeper in my mouth, a fractured tooth. I made a quick discovery. You *can* talk with your face imbedded in three pounds of ice and a Cannon bath towel. I needed one thing: I called my previous dentist, 75 miles away.

"Happy New Year from Dr. Floss! Keep smiling in 1979." There was nobody home. So I followed the answering service instructions and dialed his associate. *"Happy New Year! Go to*

the emergency room."

I called offices in two bordering states and picked up long-distance referrals, good advice, and five more Happy New Years. They apparently thought I was having a little New Year's celebration all my own:

"Eyeth neeth thoo theee thuh thenthist." (I need to see the dentist.)

"Eyeth hathd annn **ath-uh-denth!***"* (I've had an accident!)

"AAATH - UHHHH - DENNNTH."

Note: To approximate this exact pronunciation, imagine one dozen hot, melted marshmallows stuffed—all at once—into your mouth. Now say, "accident."

Finally, there is one name left in the phone book. (I start with Z and work my way backwards.) The first listing: Brandenburg, Charles Lawrence, Jr., DDS; Rising Sun, MD. A name I do not want to call. (At this point, I'm hurting and scared. Mentally, I'm several pints short of a gallon of milk.) God, help me.

CHARLES: There hasn't been a Charles on this side of the Atlantic since Lindbergh left for Paris. He's got to be *old.* BRANDENBURG: So he's old, and European? If nobody can understand *me* today, and I can't understand *him*, what's the point? RISING SUN. And he lives here. With me, and the cows. In Cowland.

What kind of dentist lives in this one-light, one-store, seventeen-thousand-head-of-Holsteins town? No dentist I want to know.

I redial the previous listing in the book. *"HAP-PY NEW YEAR!"* They're sympathetic; they're ready to help. And they're 40 miles away. So here goes nothing: Six-five-eight....

"Doctor Brandenburg's office."

"Eyeth hathd annn **ath-uh-denth.**"

"You've had an accident? Oh, my dear. You should come in immediately, Doctor Brandenburg will want to see you right away."

Yes, Virginia, there is a God.

In the office of C.L. Brandenburg, Jr., DDS, I had my mouth examined, my teeth x-rayed, and my pain treated. But good dental medicine did not make it any easier to eat—my own words. Even when we can't speak, the fearful thoughts we craft in our minds cripple us. If desperation had not driven me beyond my fear, what would that fear have cost me? At the very least, a fine dentist. And two beloved friends and mentors. Over the months of my mother's dying and my father's isolating sorrow, Larry and Libby Brandenburg took me from the dental chair and pulled me into their hearts.

Twenty-two Decembers have passed. My husband, my front tooth, and I live comfortably in the Pacific Northwest. John is a fine tenor, his younger brother, Peter, is the family percussionist, and Lucy Ricardo (a red-headed hound), our backyard baritone. Nobody plays the flute.

My "parents" are flying home this afternoon from Europe, where they celebrated their anniversary. Normally, Larry and Libby spend their vacation time in Third World nations, treating the poorest, forgotten people of the world. At home, they care for his patients, their marriage of 50 years, and the children of their six sons and daughters. And scattered among a handful of Brandenburg "adoptees," you'll find me.

s I close this simple letter, it's both late and early. The sound of my grandmother's clock rises up the stairs, chimes striking midnight. It's June 17, 2001. Happy Father's Day, Larry! You're so far away. You know, I haven't darkened the threshold of your office in years, because I'm not your patient anymore. But that's okay.

I'm still your daughter. ❤

—S.G. Cooley

11

BEYOND DENTISTRY

Everybody can be great...
because anybody can serve.
You don't have to have a college degree to
serve. You don't have to make your subject
and verb agree to serve. You only need a
heart full of grace. A soul generated by love.

—Dr. Martin Luther King, Jr.

We Care

We dwell in the shelter of one another.

—Irish Proverb

ygienists care about people—their oral health, their diets, and their hygiene habits. But just how far does our caring go? Does it extend beyond our dental chairs? Would we still care about a person if he or she wasn't our patient?

It was 1979, and I was practicing dental hygiene at an Army hospital in Wurzburg, Germany. The dental clinic was on the second floor. My room had a bird's-eye view of the helicopter pad where people were Med-Evaced in for treatment. While I was discussing brushing technique with a patient one February morning, a chopper touched down. We watched as three nurses carrying an oxygen tank and IV bags whisked a man on a gurney into the ER below me. I said a little prayer for the unfortunate soul as I did for all incoming guests at our facility.

At lunch that day, the hospital mess hall was buzzing with the report of a truck accident. A two-and-a-half-ton Army transport carrying soldiers to a field exercise had skidded on the ice and careened down an embankment. There was only one survivor—the person who had been flown in that morning. He was in the intensive care unit with extensive injuries. The doctors didn't know if he was going to make it.

"He must feel so alone," I thought out loud as I stirred my tea.

"I'll bet he does," said a nurse at my table. "His commanding officer came in for a brief visit and then left to deal with all those fatalities, notifying next of kin. The rest of this soldier's unit is still on maneuvers and can't get away to see him. His family is in the States, and he has no one right now."

I went back to work feeling deep empathy for this soldier, this person I'd never met. I imagined the panic he must have felt going over that embankment and the fear for his life as it hung in the balance. I worked that Friday afternoon with a nagging question in my mind: "Why don't I go up and see him? No," I thought, "He wasn't *my* patient." That didn't change the fact that I still cared about his wellbeing.

After my last appointment that Friday afternoon, I ran upstairs to the ICU just above the dental clinic. A nurse curtly informed me that "family only" were allowed to visit. Since he was black and I was white, any explanation I might offer wasn't going to fly. But recognizing that her patient had no family here, the nurse softened her attitude, rules were bent, and she let me stay.

I tiptoed to the soldier's bedside. He was a mass of wires and tubes connected to blinking and whirring machines. "Internal injuries," the nurse said. His eyes were closed, and I didn't know if he could hear me; but I stayed for a while and spoke reassuring and encouraging words to him. He didn't make a sound or twitch a muscle. With tears in my eyes, I left, promising to return on Monday.

I kept my promise; and this time the soldier was awake. Because the tube in his throat made it nearly impossible to speak, he was given a pad and pen to write with. He wrote that God had spared him; and he thanked me for my prior visit. I was amazed to learn he had heard me. I told him that I was praying for him and would continue until he was well again. I could see he was still in a lot of pain, needing constant medication to ease his suffering. Both he and his nurses seemed grateful for my visit. He was a soldier fighting for his life and needed all the support he could get.

Two days later, I arrived at the ICU to find his bed empty.

"His injuries were too severe," the nurse told me. "At this facility, we're not equipped to deal with such extensive internal injuries. He had to be moved."

I left the ICU thinking I'd never know what happened to that patient. A week passed, then a month. I lost track of time, but I prayed for him often.

pring arrived. I had just finished setting up for my next patient when a deep voice greeted me from the doorway. I looked up to see a tall black soldier standing there, smiling.

"The nurse in ICU told me you worked here," he said. "They just released me from the hospital in Karlsruhe. It's been rough, but you'll never know how much your visits meant to me," he said, "especially that first day in ICU. I really thought I was going to die. I never felt so alone. It was good to know that somebody cared. I told my commanding officer I had some unfinished business here, but I really just came back to say thank you."

We just can't help ourselves; hygienists care about *people*. ♥

—Joanne Iannone Sheehan, RDH

Oklahoma Healing

y parents gave this poem to my husband and me shortly after I had suffered a miscarriage in our first pregnancy. Even though the poem did not hold all the answers to our questions about "Why," it was an enormous comfort to us both. I tucked the poem away, and reflect on it from time to time as I deal with life's challenges.

My Life Is Like a Weaving

My life is like a weaving
between my God and me.
I do not choose the colors
He works steadily.

Sometimes He weaves sorrow
and I in foolish pride
forget He sees the upper,
and I, the underside.

Not till the loom is silent
and shuttles cease to fly
will God unroll the canvas
and explain the reason why
the dark threads are as needful
in the skillful Weaver's hand
as the threads of gold and silver
in the pattern He has planned.

—Grant Colfax Tullar
American hymnist (1869-1950)

After the April 19, 1995, bombing of the Alfred P. Murrah Federal Building here in Oklahoma City, I had an overwhelming desire to share a copy of this poem with my patients John and Gloria Taylor. The Taylors lost their daughter, Teresa, to this tragedy. Several office visits with them went by while the poem had lain in my drawer in the operatory.

As much as I wanted to give it to them, I didn't want to intrude on the grief they were experiencing. I knew they had already received many condolence cards and the emotional support of numerous friends and relatives; I just didn't feel anything I had to say could alleviate the pain of their loss. Then I remembered that this is exactly how my parents had felt about my miscarriage until they found the poem that said *everything* to them—and eventually to my husband and me. So I decided I needed to find the appropriate opportunity to share it with the Taylors.

Before I knew it, it was time for Gloria to come in for another dental appointment. To my surprise, she arrived at the office carrying a rolled-up piece of canvas. She explained that it was a weaving, a cross-stitching of an angel that her daughter

Teresa had begun for her as a Christmas gift. Immediately I realized this was absolutely the perfect time to give Gloria my poem.

As she held it, I looked over her shoulder and we read the verses together. Of course, we were both moved to tears and shared a warm hug afterward. Gloria took the poem home and has since had it mounted. "My Life Is Like a Weaving" now occupies a place over the mantel on the Taylor fireplace just below her late daughter's weaving of an angel. It is a wonderful reminder to them of the love and grace of God that He shares with us all, even when we cannot seem to find it. ❤

—April Klepper, RDH

Nicky

Three things in human life are important:
The first is to be kind.
The second is to be kind.
And the third is to be kind.

—Henry James

hen I graduated as a dental hygienist over ten years ago, one of the things I was unprepared for was the extremely private things people would tell me during their cleanings. I was exposed to the intimate details of messy divorces, childbirth, or, sometimes, the latest town gossip. Although I found this aspect of my work psychologically uncomfortable, I felt sincere empathy for the patients' situations and—while cleaning their teeth—offered any advice I thought might be of help.

Eight years ago, a woman named Nicole came into our practice with a broken front tooth. When I asked what had caused the problem, she said she had fallen on her way home from work. She also explained that the accident had occurred two months earlier. When asked why she had waited so long to have it fixed, she said it was because she had been so busy of late. As is the case with many of my patients, we chatted throughout the appointment.

Nicole had not been to the office in a number of years, so I had to reschedule her to complete the procedure. We decided to finish her cleaning and fix the broken tooth on the same day a couple of weeks later. Before she left, she asked me to let the receptionist know she would pay the bill in full—with cash—the next time she came in. Under no circumstances were we to send the bill to her home. She left with an estimate of how much the total cost of her treatment would be. Although her request seemed strange, neither the receptionist nor I gave it much thought at the time.

It was during the second appointment when Nicole confessed that her tooth had been broken while her husband was beating her. She had waited to come in for treatment because she had to allow time for the black eye she had sustained in the same beating to heal. She further explained that her husband felt sorry afterwards and had offered to pay to have the tooth fixed. That was why she didn't want us to send the bill home. This way she could not only get the tooth fixed, she could also have a badly needed cleaning—a procedure her husband would not permit because he thought it cost too much money. I also learned that Nicole was *not* employed, contrary to what she had told me on her first visit.

I was shocked and more than a little bewildered to learn that she was still living with this man. When I questioned her a bit further, Nicole told me that he didn't mean to hurt her; he was just under a lot of stress at work. She went on to say that although he had done this before, it was usually her fault that he hit her. She was always doing things wrong!

Well, it didn't take a rocket scientist to realize what was going on. I gave Nicole the name and office number of another patient of mine that worked at a shelter for abused women. I also tried to share with her what little I knew about spousal abuse. Nicole was not prepared to listen and told me she didn't consider herself to be a battered wife. Although I continued with that dental practice for two more years before graduating from university, getting married, and moving to a new city, Nicole did not come in for another appointment during that time.

t was eight years before I heard from Nicole again; and the circumstances surrounding our next contact were most unusual. The stage was set when a girlfriend of mine invited me to a play at the local college where I taught part time. The performance—a fundraiser for the women's shelter, Haven House—was a series of monologues dealing with contemporary women's issues. At one point, when the featured speaker discussed the abuse of a Bosnian woman, I thought again of Nicole and wondered how she might be doing. Although my curiosity would soon be resolved, its satisfaction had no direct relationship to my attendance at the play. The timing of the play was merely a coincidence—I think.

A couple of weeks later, I received an envelope at work from a woman named "Nicky" who lived in another town some distance away. Though I had no idea who Nicky was, I was quite accustomed to receiving mail related to college business from people I didn't know. Inside the envelope was a three-page letter from Nicole. She told me about her life during the years since we had last seen each other. She divorced her abusive first husband and later married a very nice man who both loved and respected her. She told me how she had had to go through a lot of counseling and soul-searching to become the person she was now—the person she was proud to be! As a symbol of her transformation, she changed her name to Nicky—after all, she had become *a totally new person!*

I was so fascinated to learn what Nicole had been through that I didn't even think about why she was writing to me. At the end of her letter, she explained that the changes in her life began the last time she sat in my dental chair. She thanked me profusely for the advice I had given her about the women's shelter! I was humbled to learn that she had thought of me almost daily as "the person who woke her up" from the nightmare of her life. She went on to say that she had thought often about contacting me but didn't know how. Finally, she got in touch with my mother who still lives in the town where I grew up.

Since receiving Nicole/Nicky's letter, I have spoken to her many times on the phone. I have a newfound appreciation for the fact that a little human compassion—and plain old listening—can really change people's lives. I have Nicky to thank for that new awareness. It is nice to hear that she is happy and healthy today, and it's heartwarming for me to know that I played a small—very small—part in it! ♥

—Mandy Hayre-Dhasi, RDH

Cradling People in My Lap

There is more hunger for love and appreciation
in this world than there is for bread.

—Mother Teresa

ost dental chairs include a movable headpiece that can be adjusted for the comfort of each patient. When a patient's teeth are to be cleaned—a procedure known as a prophylaxis or "prophy" in dental-talk—the back of the chair is reclined. This places the headpiece in a position just above the lap of the attending dental professional who is seated in a separate chair next to the patient's head.

Recently, someone asked me what I do for a living. I told them that, as a professional registered dental hygienist, I cradle people in my lap all day. While I treat my patients, they are in a most vulnerable position; and I have the wonderful opportunity to nurture their beings. At the same time, I have the honor of making their smile a little brighter—and their health a little better—by cleaning their teeth.

My education, training, and life experience afford me the opportunity to touch hundreds of lives in a positive manner each year. I can reach people and touch them in a way that few are ever granted. Each patient affords me the unique opportunity to learn, to grow, and to understand the world just a little more. I love hearing about trips to other countries, seeing pictures of patient's families, and sharing recipes that expand my culinary skills. What I love most of all, though, is the patients who teach me about life. Cora was such a patient.

It had been a long and challenging day, and a little voice inside me warned that it was only going to get worse! This was confirmed when I looked at the schedule and realized that my last appointment would be with my most difficult patient. Cora entered the operatory with her usual sour face—the same one she always brought with her. The way she left her coat on and sat in the chair with her arms folded, it was as if she wanted to shut out the whole world. She answered my questions with one-word grunts as I asked about her day and if there was anything exciting, new, or different in her life. So many times before, I had tried to get through to Cora—I'd used everything from humor to music—but nothing seemed to work. She was just downright rude!

On a typical appointment, Cora would turn her head away from me every time I tried to clean her teeth. She gagged whenever I tried to enter her mouth. She always acted as though I was causing her great pain in spite of my efforts to be as gentle as possible. It was apparent that she really didn't want to be there with me. I often wondered why she bothered to come back; she clearly wasn't interested in anything I had to say and took none of my oral health suggestions to heart.

That late afternoon when I began her prophy, I gently touched her face to turn her head toward me. She flinched, and I immediately saw fear in her eyes. A light came on for me—I finally had a clue as to how to get through to Cora. I put down my prophy tools—placing them in the tray in front of my patient—and proceeded to tell her of some volunteer work I was doing at a battered women's shelter. I was collecting used clothing and asked my patients to bring in any donations they might want to make. I told Cora how rewarding it was for me to be able to help in this way.

Tears flowed down her cheeks as she shared with me the story of her mother who didn't have a battered women's shelter to go to when Cora was a child. We cried together as I told her of the resources now available to people who are suffering abuse. It was then that Cora revealed what I had begun to suspect—she was being abused in her *own* relationship. Although I didn't finish cleaning her teeth that afternoon, I have to say that this was the most productive and satisfying day of my career.

hat appointment turned out to be Cora's first step toward recovery. Although she has thanked me countless times since, it is I who am indebted to her. She taught me so much! She trusted me enough to share the most vulnerable part of her life. A bright young woman, Cora got the help she needed. She has since become a model dental patient—no longer fearful of my gentle touch when she allows me the privilege of cradling her in my lap. ♥

—Noel Brandon-Kelsch, RDH

Blessed Event

Those who loved you and were helped by you
will remember you.
So carve your name on hearts and not on marble.

—C.H. Spurgeon

hile working as a dental hygienist in a large midwestern city, I met a registered nurse in her mid-thirties named Dianne. During one of our initial hourlong therapy appointments, she told me she was married but had no children. Something in our dialog made me think she wanted to have children very much. Dianne was an articulate and interesting woman, and we developed an immediate rapport. During the course of her therapy, we had many nice conversations, and every now and then she would bring up the fact that she had no children.

Since Dianne had mentioned the subject so often, I finally decided to pursue the matter further and asked if she might have a fertility problem.

"Oh, no!" she laughed, "It's not that at all! It's just that Steve and I are so busy with our careers and lives that we...uh...uh...just don't have time to *do it!*"

I laughed and said, "Well, I can't help you with *that* one!" Moments later, the radio in my operatory began to play the

Percy Sledge song "When a Man Loves a Woman." I stopped
cleaning her teeth and turned up the volume.

I said, "Dianne, listen to this. It's one of the most romantic
songs I know. Get this CD, and play it for your husband. I
guarantee you'll find the time." We both laughed and enjoyed
the rest of that great song.

Several months passed, and one day Dianne came in for a
follow-up cleaning appointment. I was reviewing her health
and medical history when I sensed she was very excited about
something.

"Well, aren't you going to ask me?" she blurted out.

"Ask you what?" I said.

"I'm five months pregnant—the song—I bought the CD. It
worked!" She beamed at me. Since Dianne was so tall and
slender, her pregnancy barely showed and I was completely
surprised.

We giggled like two schoolgirls during the rest of her
appointment while we discussed Lamaze classes, baby names,
and other "baby stuff." Dianne was by then on a six-month
recall, and I made her promise to bring in baby pictures at her
next checkup. She did much better than that.

Six months later, she showed up with Lindsey, her beautiful,
healthy, two-month-old daughter. Dianne introduced the
infant to me and told her, "This is the lady who helped us have
you." She gave me a lot of the credit, and I admit it felt great
when I saw how much happiness this child had brought into
her life.

t was some time later when Dianne's husband,
Steve, showed up at our office as a new patient. I
was so excited to meet the final member of the
happy trio that I said, "Hi, I'm the woman who
helped you get pregnant. No, no, I mean...."

"You must be Sherrie," he said, interrupting my embarrassment. "Dianne told me I had to meet you. And, hey, the

song was great!" He gave me a thumbs-up sign and mouthed the word "Thanks."

Sometimes in dentistry, our most rewarding moments have nothing at all to do with teeth. ♥

—Sherrie Frame, RDH

Puppy Therapy

*There is no therapy in all the world
quite like a puppy licking your face.*

—Charles Schulz

hile we were having our morning dental office
meeting to discuss the day's cancellations, the
phone rang. A patient called to see if there were
any last-minute openings so that he could have his
teeth cleaned.

Our caller, a kindly minister, came in to see me at 11 AM.
He had just finished visiting a family that belonged to his
church. The minister sadly told me of their three-year-old
daughter, Chelsea, who had leukemia and explained how
tough her illness was on the whole family. It was especially
hard on Josh, Chelsea's seven-year-old brother. It seemed Josh
had become a very sad and withdrawn big brother.

As I thought about the plight of this family, I recalled a conversation I had had with my teenage daughter, Sandy, that very
morning. Sandy was worried about finding good homes for all of
our new puppies. I told Sandy about the minister's story later
that evening. When she looked up at me, we both knew that
Josh had to have one of our puppies. I then called the minister
and asked if he thought the family would accept a beautiful
AKC-registered Golden Retriever puppy as a gift. He seemed
excited about the idea and said he'd talk to them about it.

A few days later, the minister returned to the dental office to see me. He had spoken with Josh and Chelsea's parents and learned that neither one of them had ever owned a pet. Since they were concerned about their daughter's compromised immune system, they decided to consult with Chelsea's physician before considering our offer. The doctor told them that a puppy would be ideal for the entire family and would pose no threat to Chelsea's immune system.

Over the next couple of years, Sandy and I received many touching letters from Josh's mom. She always told us about Josh's enthusiasm for living. Every day, he'd run home from school and fly like a bolt of lightning through the house into the backyard where his precious dog and best companion eagerly awaited his return. Josh even built a doghouse with spare lumber he gathered from the neighborhood.

The most touching of all the letters had enclosed with it a family portrait—dog and all. Chelsea had grown so much. She was a beautiful little girl with long, dark flowing curls and the biggest smile. The letter said that her leukemia had gone into remission.

I showed the letter to Sandy and asked, "Isn't it wonderful?"

My daughter smiled and said, "Yes, it sure is. But Mom, do you have any more patients that know someone who needs a puppy? We're expecting another litter." ❤

—Deborah D. Landis, RDH

Eighteen Months

Oh heart, if someone should say to you
that the soul perishes like the body,
answer that the flower perishes
but the seed remains.
This is the law of God.

—Kahlil Gibran

y patient's name was Rose, and she came in to see me every three months to have her teeth cleaned. Due to arthritis, her homecare—regular brushing and flossing—was not always what it should have been. This neglect was reflected in the condition of her gums, which were not in very good shape. During one visit, Rose questioned me about a small growth that had appeared on her palate. One look and I knew that it was a most suspicious lesion. I immediately asked the dentist to examine her, and of course, he referred Rose to an oral surgeon right away.

A biopsy revealed that the growth in Rose's mouth was a cancerous tumor traceable to an old breast malignancy she had had years earlier. Since this is quite uncommon, a few more biopsies were performed to confirm the diagnosis. Subsequently, half of her palate and upper teeth were surgically removed. When she returned in about a year to have her remaining teeth cleaned, the first thing I noticed was a fresh growth in her mouth. I immediately suspected what it was but didn't have the heart to tell her. Instead, I talked about what she had been through, commiserated with her, and just tried to make her feel good about herself.

I then asked the dentist to reexamine my patient as the lesion obviously took priority over teeth cleaning. He again referred her to the oral surgeon, and unfortunately, our worst fears were confirmed. Rose lived only another six months, but she was kept comfortable and clean in the care of her loving husband.

Shortly after Rose's demise, I ran into her husband in the bank. Although my impression of him had always been that he was not an affectionate person, he came over and hugged me dearly saying, "Jane, I owe you a *huge* debt of gratitude."

"Why, Morton?" I asked.

"If it wasn't for you, I wouldn't have had my precious Rose for the extra 18 months that I did!" Of course we both had tears in our eyes, and I thanked him for sharing his feelings with me. Is it any wonder that I *still* love my job—even after 37 years in the profession? ❤

—Jane Weiner, RDH

Golfer's Last Wish

*What a beautiful place a golf course is. From the meanest
country pasture to the Pebble Beaches and St. Andrews of the
world, a golf course is to me a holy ground. I feel God in the
trees and grass and flowers, in the rabbits and the birds and
the squirrels, in the sky and the water. I feel that I am home.*

—Harvey Penick

avid came in for a routine dental exam and was
asked if there were any changes in his health history.
A very sad look clouded his face as he said, "I've
been diagnosed with prostate cancer, and the prognosis is poor. But I'm a very lucky man; I have a family that
loves me, a beautiful home, and a decent golf handicap."
David told me he had been all over the country looking for a
cure, but not one of the doctors had offered any hope. Because
his prognosis had been so poor, some experimental treatment
with hormones had been attempted—to no avail. He joked,
"My wife and I got to have hot flashes together."

During a subsequent visit, the conversation turned to his
cancer, and I asked him a pointed question: "Is there anything
you would like to do before you die?"

Without hesitation, he said, "Play golf at the Augusta
National Golf Club." David knew many people, but Georgia's
Augusta National—home of the Masters Tournament—is by
invitation only, and he had not been able to find anyone who

knew a member. I smiled at his request; since I'm not a golfer, to me an iron is something you press clothes with and a driver is a person who operates a motor vehicle.

I decided I had to help this man play golf at Augusta before he died. I knew that our banker was from Augusta, so I called him and cried as I explained my patient's situation. My friend said he would see what he could do. Several days later, the banker got back to me with the news that all had been arranged.

One of the best phone calls I've ever made was to tell Dave to pack his clubs because he had a tee time at the Augusta National Golf Club. His excitement was contagious; and he joked over the fact that a non-golfer like me had helped arrange what his New Jersey golf buddies believed to be impossible. He later explained that—due to business commitments—he planned to fly down the morning of his tee time. Fortunately, I was able to convince him to reschedule his meetings because Augusta was the opportunity of a lifetime. I urged him to go the day before his tee time in case his flight was delayed, clubs got lost, or some other obstacle reared its ugly head.

Dave's round of golf at the Augusta National Golf Club was everything he had hoped it would be. The experience was made even sweeter by the fact that people who didn't even know him had volunteered their time. Helping Dave was the most selfless thing I've ever done; and I was thrilled to have had a role in making his dream come true.

 everal years have passed since then, and David's health has stabilized. Every spring, I now make time to watch the televised Masters Tournament at the Augusta National Golf Club. And when I see the azaleas blooming in the background, I'm reminded that David has enjoyed one more year. ❤

—Allyson K. Hurley, DDS, MAGD, AACD

12

OUTSIDE
THE BOX

And life is what we make of it.
Always has been.
Always will be.

—Grandma Moses

Today Is a Gift

Be courageous.
It's one of the only places left uncrowded.

—Anita Roddick

oesn't it bother you that one of your pupils is dilated?" is a question I am asked from time to time. My response is always the same: "No. Not at all." Every day when I look in the mirror, I am reminded that today is a gift and that I am blessed to be here. And since today is a gift, I want to make sure that I can look back on this day—and every day—and say, "I am so glad that I did...." rather than look back with regret and say, "I wish I had done...."

I *do* have one pupil that is fixed and dilated. It doesn't track too well either. When I look up or down, things are double. "That's why God gave you a neck, Cathy," stated my neurosurgeon, "so that you can move your head up or down, get focused, and then take the next step." And that daily reminder is the only remaining after-effect of a horse accident that nearly took my life, but instead, has become a source of inspiration.

August 1. Hot. Dry. Ground as hard as concrete. That describes the condition of the earth on that blistering summer day when my daughter, niece, and nephew asked me to take them on a horseback ride across our ranch in southern Oklahoma. We raise Registered American Quarter Horses on our ranch, so I was pleased the kids wanted to ride that day and was more than happy to orchestrate and participate in this trail ride.

The young man who works with us on the ranch helped me gather the horses and groom, saddle, and bridle them. I was going to ride our stallion that day, but upon getting him out of his stall found that he was a bit sore from the previous day's activities. So I gave him a day of rest and chose to ride Especial Doll, one of our best "show" mares. She was a bit skittish by nature, but I had ridden and shown her many times and *thought* I was familiar with her temperament.

Once we maneuvered through the gate to the pasture, I helped the kids "get on board," then mounted Especial Doll. I usually saddle and bridle my own horse, but that day, my assistant had offered to do this while I helped the kids. I saw him put a bit into her mouth that was different than the one she was used to, but I didn't think she would mind since she was a seasoned veteran.

Wrong! Once the kids were mounted, I put my foot into the stirrup and climbed aboard. I picked up the reins and "checked" my mare to let her know we were ready to go. When she felt that unfamiliar bit in her mouth, she threw her head between her legs and started running backwards. She stopped. Planted herself. Reared up and fell over. When she fell over backwards, so did I. The last thing I remembered for the subsequent five weeks was the sensation of kicking my feet out of the stirrups. And it's a good thing. Unrestrained and frightened, the horse ran a couple of miles across the ranch through trees, brush, and rough terrain. Had my foot stuck in that stirrup, I would have been torn to shreds.

The moment the back of my head hit that concrete-like earth I went into a coma. And so, the information I will now share is the recounting of events as told to me by others.

The kids ran to the barn, hysterical. Anxiously, they told my assistant about the accident, and he immediately called an ambulance from a small town five miles away. The ambulance arrived, and I was transported to the hands of a physician who had been an emergency doctor in Vietnam. He knew what to do in the case of a massive head injury and began administering appropriate medications.

My dentist husband, John, was in another hospital some 20 miles away and had a three-year-old child under general anesthesia and had 14 teeth prepped. My attending physician had him called out of the operating room and—over the phone—told him what had happened. "John, I'm sorry to tell you this, but Cathy has been in a terrible accident. She is in a coma. She is paralyzed. Her pupils are fixed and dilated. She is breathing. But, I can't tell you whether or not I will be able to keep her alive. If I do stabilize her, I have to get her to Oklahoma City (which was one and a half hours away), and I have to get her into the hands of a neurosurgeon. Give me the name of the hospital and doctor you choose, then I have to get back in there with her."

John gave him the necessary information and went back into the operating room and finished the treatment on the child. When the dental procedures were completed, the physicians told him they would bring the child back around from anesthesia. The child's parents, of course, agreed.

People now ask how in the world John was able to complete the treatment on that little girl. Who knows? He thinks an angel came down to lend a helping hand. So do I.

Fear of the unknown is powerful and can be traumatic. John discovered this truism as he followed the ambulance in a separate vehicle. My attending physician had cancelled his afternoon patients and had ridden in the ambulance with me. But there was no communication between the ambulance and John during that seemingly endless trip.

John says that he cried uncontrollably the entire way. He told me, "I didn't know what I would face when they opened the back doors of that ambulance. I didn't know if you would be alive or dead. I was so afraid that the doctor would step out of that ambulance and say, 'I'm sorry, John, she didn't make it.' I knew you were paralyzed and that you had extensive brain damage. I was prepared to take care of you in a vegetative state for the rest of your life. But, I couldn't stand to think about raising our two kids alone. I wanted you to be their mom, Cath. I couldn't bear the thought of living without you."

The doors of the ambulance did open to an alive patient—but one who was "gone." For five weeks, I floated in and out of a comatose state. I remember nothing about those five weeks. When I began to come around and the doctors felt that it was safe for me to be dismissed, they sent me to my parents' home for a couple of months of recuperation.

Two neurosurgeons were on my case. One had practiced 35 years and one had practiced ten years: 45 years of neurosurgery! They said that I had the worst concussion throughout my entire brain that they had ever seen. I had third, fifth, and seventh cranial nerve damage. The cranial nerves are the only nerves of the body that do not regenerate. They told us that on the CAT scans, they couldn't tell whether the nerves were severed or bruised. If the nerves were severed, I would never function again, they informed us. If the nerves were bruised, they thought I might have some healing, but would never function normally again.

We left the hospital with little or no encouragement.

People asked me how I recovered. I couldn't see. Couldn't walk. Couldn't think.

I, personally, believe that I had powerful help from above. I have a strong, loving family and a circle of friends who were there through the thick and the thin of the accident and the long year of rehabilitation. I had spent a lifetime focusing on the positive, being a goal setter, and believing in possibility. So, when the conscious part of me was gone, and the doctors said that I would never function again, the subconscious part of me had been well fed. The subconscious part of me said, "Oh, yeah? Stand back and watch." Excellent medicine and pharmaceuticals combined with the power of a Higher Being and a positive mental attitude.

I am no different than anyone else. I don't have any more

gifts than anyone else. I've just had the privilege of being thrown real hard on my head, and was poignantly shown that I could get back up, put my foot back in the stirrup, and climb back into the saddle again. The physicians can't explain it. But, they don't have to. They know that miracles do happen— every day.

 f you haven't already been thrown on your head by one of life's many challenges, you will be. Someone may leave you, and you can't imagine how you will be able to go on. You may become ill or have a physical ailment or accident that changes your life. A child may break your heart. You may experience financial woe. There are challenges throughout life that seem unbearable. But God will never give you more than you can handle. And if you face your challenges and learn from each and every one of them, you will be able to put your foot back into the stirrup and get back in the saddle. And when you do, you will be stronger on the other side.

The dilated pupil. Does it bother me? Not a bit! It remains—today and every day—a reminder of the fact that today is a gift. For me—and for you. Cherish the gift. ♥

—Cathy Jameson, PhD

Taking a Bite
Out of Crime

t was a terrible day! I woke up late, so I didn't have time to take my morning run or even chew over the morning news. There were no leftovers to enjoy for breakfast, and worst of all I had a toothache like you wouldn't believe. Fortunately, I had an afternoon dental appointment scheduled with Dr. Robertson. I could hardly wait. My partner, Mitch, offered to take me to the appointment, so he picked me up at my house. First, we headed to the police station.

Mitch and I have been police partners for about two years and get along extremely well. Although he still considers me a rookie and usually sends *me* in to do all the dirty work, Mitch and I have recently been featured in our local newspaper as having a "nose" for crime. Most of our assignments involve drug trafficking investigations and manhunts. We work as a team, but I seem to be the one that always ends up chasing the bad guys.

Once we arrived at the station we picked up our assignment, grabbed some snacks, and headed out into the city. I didn't feel like doing anything; my tooth had taken over my entire life. All of my teeth were in bad condition and seemed to be falling out. It felt like I had used my teeth to cut through a chain link fence. I had never taken care of my teeth, and now I was paying the price. Furthermore, I had never even been to a dentist, so you can understand why I was more than a little nervous.

The morning passed quickly, and soon it was time to visit Dr. Robertson's office. When we arrived, they called my name and I was given a tour of the entire place. Dr. Robertson seated me in a comfortable chair and began his examination. He found that I needed a crown to replace one of my broken teeth. Mitch confirmed that this was the best option for me; and while I had no say in the matter, I was more than ready to be out of pain.

The procedure began, and I was relieved to discover that Dr. Robertson was very gentle. No longer nervous, I actually became interested in everything Dr. Robertson and his staff were doing. In fact, I was *so* relaxed I fell asleep. When I awoke, Dr. Robertson was washing his hands and talking with Mitch. I suddenly realized that the crown must be finished and that my tooth wasn't hurting anymore. I became so excited I jumped up, ran over to Dr. Robertson, and began licking him all over his face. I didn't know how I was going to repay him, but I was determined to do something. I wanted to let everyone in the world know how much better a dentist can make you feel!

As Mitch drove me back to my kennel, all I could think about was how thankful I was to have met Dr. Robertson and his staff. How fortunate humans are to have the opportunity to go see their dentists when they have toothaches. The news of my experience spread throughout the community. I even got my picture in the local human newspaper because it seems that most dentists aren't given the opportunity to work on us dogs. Except for Dr. Robertson, that is; he has helped many of my canine buddies in the North Little Rock, Arkansas, K-9 Corps. After my treatment, I felt like myself again: back chasing the bad guys, sniffing out drugs, and eating tons of leftovers.

I'll never forget my toothache—or my experience at Dr. Robertson's. Dentists can make your world a much better place. So I urge you to take advantage of the opportunity you have as humans to see your dentist, not only when you're in pain, but at your six-month checkups too! Thank you again, Dr. Robertson. ♥

—Kay Nine Cop
Submitted by Christy Ellis King, RDH, RDA
In Memory of William R. Robertson, DDS

Bomb Squad

I don't make jokes.
I just watch the government and report the facts.

—Will Rogers

 have been in dental practice for a long time and have many wonderful memories of a lot of good, down-to-earth patients, one of whom is Mary Pat. Mary Pat first came to our office in 1974, and we have been kidding each other and telling stories ever since. She is now a well-known, highly respected Federal judge, noted for her sense of humor and fairness. While we have the utmost admiration for each other, we still have a lot of fun. The story she told me during a recent dental visit tops all others. Even if I wanted to, I couldn't possibly add to it, or even exaggerate any aspects. This is exactly the way it happened.

It seems that Judge Mary Pat Thynge was hearing a case that involved a dentist. After the trial, the dentist—also a woman—engaged Judge Thynge in conversation on several topics, one of which involved a unique electric toothbrush now on the market that has proven highly effective with her patients. The dentist promised to send one to the judge as a professional courtesy.

A short time later, while the Judge was in a mediation session with some Secret Service agents, she was informed that there was a package for her in the mailroom...a *suspicious* package.

The return address was unfamiliar, and X rays of the package cast serious concerns as to whether this was, in fact, a *bomb*. Upon further investigation, she was able to determine that this was the electric toothbrush sent to her by the appreciative dentist. Part of the confusion was due to the fact that the shipment had originated with the dentist's husband who had a different last name.

However, the wheels of our government agencies had already been set in motion and could not be reversed—or even stopped! From her chambers, Judge Thynge watched as a large helicopter hovered overhead carrying a huge metal box swinging at the end of a chain. The "bomb-sniffing" dogs were not impressed with the package and seemed to be asking each other, "Just what are we doing here?" The "Michelin Man" in his padded suit was there also. Next, the package was shot with a gun—in order to explode the "bomb." Nothing happened. I asked Mary Pat what was left of the "mystery package." She smiled and replied that some of the replaceable brush heads were salvaged.

I would like to now report that the Federal courthouse is safe, 9th Street (which was closed during this "bomb scare") is again open, and operations are back to normal. The "bomb" was placed in an ordinary trashcan, and the bomb squad can once again rest easy. So, if you send any package to the courthouse, make sure you either place it in a clear plastic box or—at the very least—a bulletproof container.

By the way, Mary Pat informed me that the dentist sent her another electric toothbrush. I forgot to ask by what means it was sent; I think I was laughing too hard. ♥

—Charles S. Horn, III, DDS

Sammy, Poor Sammy

hen the dental assistant tiptoed into the treatment room and whispered in my ear that two police detectives had come to speak with me, I mumbled an excuse to my patient, asked her to rinse her mouth, and went out to greet them.

"How can I help you, officers?" I inquired in a higher-pitched voice than the one I normally use. In fact, I seemed to recall using that particular voice when I tried to talk a traffic cop out of giving me a speeding ticket a few years back.

"Tell us what you know about Sammy Rinaldi," they demanded. Sammy, a pleasant fellow who lived alone, had been my patient for years. Recently, he had developed some sort of acute depression or psychological illness; he lost his job and became a homeless derelict. He showed up sporadically at my office looking for a handout. I always gave him a five-dollar bill and invariably begged him to let me help by getting him to a mental-health center for treatment. He always accepted the five-dollar bill but never my offer.

I notified the policemen that I had not seen Sammy in quite a while. They explained that Sammy's estranged mother had just died and had left Sammy a small fortune, and that some of Sammy's cousins had verified that a recent unidentified suicide victim was actually Sammy, their missing relative. "We need you to come to the city morgue with Sammy's dental records and do a forensic dental identification of the corpse," announced a gum-chewing officer.

The detectives drove me to a dimly lit, nondescript building. I felt like I was in a 1950s "B" movie. An associate coroner, with a discernible limp, led me to a cold room lit by a bare bulb dangling from the ceiling. I noticed a stainless steel table topped by a sheet-draped corpse.

Sammy was single, with neither siblings nor children. The table was surrounded by a gaggle of Sammy's cousins who were, presumably, his rightful heirs. A coroner's assistant, who took notes at a rapid pace as the cousins spoke, completed the gathering. "It's Sammy, poor Sammy!" cried one. "I could recognize him immediately," sobbed another. "It seems like just yesterday that I was at his christening," added a third. All were dabbing with tissues and handkerchiefs at what appeared to me to be perfectly dry eyes. They watched my movements with great suspicion.

I pulled on my gloves and tried to act with professional detachment as I set up Sammy's X rays. The assistant pulled back the sheet and explained that witnesses had seen the victim jump in front of a speeding train.

I felt like I was back in general anatomy class in dental school. The corpse's head and neck were mangled beyond recognition but did bear a superficial resemblance to Sammy Rinaldi. After examining the mouth for just a few moments, I was convinced that the corpse was *not* Sammy. This jaw contained teeth that Sammy was missing. I announced, "This is definitely *not* Sammy Rinaldi. The forensic evidence is clear and beyond any possible doubt."

The assembled cousins began muttering. "He's a quack," complained one.

"What does he know," added another.

A third cousin said nothing but stared at me malevolently while making an unmistakable slitting motion across his throat. I left the morgue hastily.

Two weeks later, a very disheveled-looking and unkempt Sammy Rinaldi showed up at my office looking for a five-dollar handout. He couldn't understand what all the excitement was about. ♥

—Jeffrey M. Galler, DDS, MAGD

Eye Teeth

Even the smallest act of kindness says "I care,"
says "You matter," says "I thought of you."

—Jenny DeVries

 have worked as a dental assistant for 41 years—
most recently at a special dental clinic at the
University of North Carolina Hospital in Chapel
Hill. At the clinic, patients often have oral surgery
before undergoing operations for serious and, in many cases,
life-threatening problems. You see the presence of infection
anywhere in the body—including the mouth—can overload
the immune system and cause severe postsurgery problems.

One time we had a patient from a rural part of North
Carolina who needed to have several teeth extracted. I noticed
that his eyeglasses were so dirty they looked like they hadn't
been cleaned in years. While the patient was in the chair, I
gave his glasses a really good cleaning.

A few weeks later, when the gentleman returned to the
clinic for some follow-up work, I asked how he had been doing
since we extracted his teeth.

"Fine!" he replied enthusiastically. "I could really see good
after I had my teeth pulled." ❤

—Betty Moss, CDA
Submitted by her son, Bill Moss

Blurred Vision

*Blessed is he who has learned to laugh at himself,
for he shall never cease to be entertained.*

—John Bowell

n preparation for cleaning the teeth of my next patient, I put on my glasses, gloves, and mask. I then proceeded to explain to her that she had periodontal disease—bleeding gums—and that she needed to be more attentive to her homecare—regular brushing and flossing. The longer I talked, the more aware I became of how queasy my stomach was starting to feel. I also noticed that my vision was beginning to blur. All the while I was talking, I wondered, "What is happening to me?"

After several minutes had passed, I realized my patient wasn't listening to a word I said. To make matters worse, she was giving me strange looks. I started to get annoyed because I was doing my best to help her health problem. My anti-periodontal disease instructions continued for several more minutes while my dizziness and nausea grew worse.

Since my patient didn't seem to care one bit about what I had to say, I decided to stop wasting my breath and begin the dental cleaning. However—since my vision was blurred—I thought it best to remove my glasses and wipe them. Only then did I realize that I had been wearing *my patient's glasses* the whole time! I examined the glasses again—looked at my patient—and then we both started laughing uncontrollably. She apologized for not concentrating on what I was saying because she couldn't figure out why I was wearing her glasses. Since then, every time she comes to my office, we both remember that day and enjoy another good laugh. ♥

—Ethel Wolff, RDH

Live the Dream

Nice, how we never get dizzy from doing good turns.
—George Bengis

ovember nights fall early in Minneapolis. It was dark by 4:30 when I finished delivering my daylong dental seminar, polishing off the session with a rock-solid close. It's impossible at a moment like that not to feel really good. An impromptu entourage followed me through the hotel corridors as I made my way toward the lobby. I stopped to talk with the conference delegates because I love people. I really do. Although the travel my speaking engagements demand is stimulating, that's not *it* for me—the people I meet make it all worthwhile.

So that moment, when my colleagues and I reached the lobby, was perfect. The payoff of the day. Standing at my left was a young dentist from St. Paul who joined the others in appraising my lecture. It was an engaging conversation. But somewhere between his appreciation and my responding comment, the voice and the face from St. Paul dissolved.... I was distracted by the sight of a formally dressed young man as he passed the registration desk and stopped at an archway.

It was the tuxedo that drew my attention—he was dressed to kill, every hair in place. His mother walked beside him, her face beaming with maternal pride. An old man strode briskly toward the couple, caught up, and touched the boy on the shoulder. The boy spun around, hesitated a moment, and then called out, "Daddy—Daddy, you made it!"

The old man melted into his son's black satin-tuxedoed arms. *"David, I wouldn't have missed your prom for anything."* I watched as a father pressed his face into his child's shoulder, reaching up with a free hand to wipe his own tears. They all embraced. The boy's twinkling eyes—huge behind bottle-thick lenses—magnified the happiness the trio shared. And David is 40 years old.

So began the parade. Young people in evening dress, youths in adult bodies: the mentally challenged. Driving through the lobby were paired wheelchairs, couples side by side. Here and there a bare head, cancer patients heading for the dance floor. Young people bright with excitement, fighting the contortions of cerebral palsy.

One by one they passed me, a fluid stream—dozens, then scores—there must have been a hundred or more. I stared at the procession in wonder, stunned by the realization that one thread tied these people together—simple joy.

But I didn't feel any *joy.* What I felt was more like sorrow, humility—*guilt!* What is it that kicks you in the guts and makes you feel guilty—for being whole? I don't know. I didn't have to know.

ix months later, I watched a sequel of Minneapolis. We were all together—my entire dental office team, my wife June, our three kids, the catering people, and the best DJ in New Jersey. In our tuxes, we looked like a wedding party at the Ritz! The room was vibrant with music. Servers wove between us, hors d'oeuvre trays glued to their fingertips. And then our first guest stepped in. Dressed for the Oscars, he escorted his date and his parents. We were told about Eric, he was 51. Then a couple in matching wheelchairs arrived. Michele from my office stepped up to greet them. "Good evening, good evening! Welcome to the Moonlight Room!" The celebration had begun.

"Hi, I'm Karen. You wanna dance?" The woman clutched at my jacket like she could break me in half—all four feet of her. She looked up into my face—and then dropped her head with a girlish grin. She didn't know—or care—who I was. Smiling at the floor, Karen whispered into my chest, *"This is the best day of my LIFE!"*

ho made this dream possible? The list is long. My practice staff contacted the Association of Retarded Citizens (ARC), and from there it grew like all good collaborations. We tried something new. And six months after Minnesota, there we were in New Jersey, watching Karen dance to the music on the best day of her life.

The ups and downs of my own life have proven to me—so many times—that *everybody* has a dream. It doesn't take an Einstein or a Charles Atlas to dream. The men and women who pull together, trying to find the stuff that dreams are made of...they don't *ask* for thanks. They *owe* their thanks. I owe *my* thanks to Karen in Bridgeton, New Jersey, and to David back in Minneapolis. *I owe them.*

What they create, I cannot make. What they give, I cannot purchase. For nobody buys a dream: you *live* it. ♥

—Steven L. Rasner, DMD, MAGD

Story Contest for the Sequel to This Book

We are planning to publish *Love Is the Best Medicine™ for Dental Patients and the Dental Team—Volume Two* in the fall of 2003 and are conducting a story contest as a means of assembling a new collection of outstanding true stories about dentistry for that edition. The contest deadline is May 1, 2003.

Four grand prizes of $1,000 each will be awarded to the author of the best story by a dentist, a dental hygienist, a dental assistant, and a dental office administrator. All others whose stories are selected for publication will receive compensation in the form of 20 copies of the book. For this compensation, authors agree to provide DMD House with the non-exclusive rights to publish their stories. For a full set of contest rules and submission deadlines for various titles, please visit our website or send us a self-addressed stamped envelope with your request.

Non-returnable submissions should be sent to:

Story Contest Editor
DMD House
29925 Rose Blossom Drive, Suite 300
Murrieta, CA 92563-4735 USA
Email: dondible@dmdhouse.net
Fax: 909.698.0180
Website: www.dmdhouse.net

All non-returnable submissions should include the name, address, phone number, and email address (if you have one) of the author. A postcard will be sent acknowledging receipt of all materials. Please keep a copy of all submissions for your files.

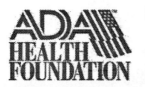 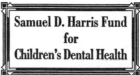

In the spirit of fostering more love in the world, a portion of the proceeds from sales of *Love Is the Best Medicine™ for Dental Patients and the Dental Team* will go to the Samuel D. Harris Fund for Children's Dental Health, a permanent endowment fund of the ADA Health Foundation. The primary objective of this program is the prevention of tooth decay and other oral diseases in children, particularly for those children whose economic status places them at greatest risk of not receiving adequate oral health education and access to preventive care.

The ADA Health Foundation is the leading national charitable organization with the primary focus of enhancing clinical dentistry and, in turn, the oral health of the American public. It accomplishes this central mission by providing funds—gathered from grants, government agencies, and private contributions—for charitable projects, awareness activities, and basic and applied dental research and educational programs.

Because of its strategic ties with the American Dental Association, the ADA Health Foundation's ability to advance clinical dentistry is greatly strengthened. Funding is provided to a wide range of philanthropic programs aimed at improving dentistry's understanding of oral diseases and increasing both access to and quality of dental care for all populations. By fostering continuous advancement in dental research, education, and access, the Foundation significantly affects the oral health of the public and the practice of dentistry.

ADA Health Foundation
Samuel D. Harris Fund for Children's Dental Health
211 E. Chicago Avenue
Chicago, IL 60611
Phone: 312.440.2547 • Fax: 312.440.3526
Email: adahf@ada.org

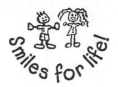

A portion of the proceeds from sales of this book will be contributed to the Smiles for Life Foundation, an organization created by the Crown Council to bless the lives of children all over North America. The Crown Council is a group of elite dental teams dedicated to building outstanding dental practices while making significant contributions to their communities. The membership of the Crown Council commissioned the Smiles for Life Foundation in 1998 as a means of giving something back to the communities where they live.

Since 1998, members of the Crown Council have taken four months each year to participate in the Smiles for Life Teeth-Whitening Campaign. During the campaign period, proceeds from all teeth-whitening are contributed to the Smiles for Life Foundation. Discus Dental contributes all of the professional whitening material and the dentists contribute the professional service so that all of the proceeds can benefit the Foundation. Since 1998, over $11,000,000 has been received by the Foundation. Those interested in participating in the annual teeth-whitening campaign are invited to call 877.4.SMILES where they will be referred to the closest participating Crown Council member. Information is also available at www.smiles4life.com.

In partnership with Garth Brooks's Teammates for Kids Foundation, Smiles for Life has made contributions to more than 100 children's charities in North America, including major contributions to the St. Jude Children's Research Hospital, the Children's Dental Center, and Steven Spielberg's Starbright Foundation.

Smiles for Life Foundation
923 E. Executive Park Drive, Suite C
Salt Lake City, UT 84117
Phone: 800.276.9658 • Fax: 801.293.8524
Website: www.smiles4life.com

Give Back A Smile™ Program

It is an unfortunate reality that more than five million people in the United States are affected by domestic violence each year. Sadly, the emotional and physical damage from domestic violence can drain the passion for life from the survivors. In 1999, the American Academy of Cosmetic Dentistry® (AACD) founded the Give Back A Smile™ program through its charitable foundation to provide those in need with a new smile. The program provides free reconstructive dental work to women and men who have had their teeth adversely affected by domestic violence. Through Give Back A Smile™, many people have had their smiles restored and their outlook on life rejuvenated.

In the spring of 2001, Give Back A Smile™ received the prestigious Award of Excellence, sponsored by the American Society of Association Executives, and the ASAE's highest distinction, the Summit Award, in the 2001 Association's Advance America Awards program. As one of only eight programs to receive the Summit Award each year, participants in the Give Back A Smile™ program are leading examples of people who care about, and are able to give help to, those in desperate need.

All AACD members are encouraged to participate in Give Back A Smile™. Doctors can gain personal satisfaction from applying their wonderful skills to a worthy cause. The AACD and the Give Back A Smile™ program clearly demonstrate that cosmetic dentistry has the ability to change lives for the better.

A portion of the proceeds from the purchase of *Love Is the Best Medicine™ for Dental Patients and the Dental Team* will be donated to the Give Back A Smile™ program. For information regarding how doctors can participate in Give Back A Smile™, visit www.aacd.com. For those interested in finding help with the Give Back A Smile™ program, call the national hotline: 800.773.GBAS (4227) or send an email to Claudia Patchen, Foundation Coordinator, at givebackasmile@aacd.com.

Donald M. Dible

In his long career as an entrepreneur and consultant, Don has produced more than 10,000 seminars and dozens of conferences. He has more than a decade of experience as a seminar and conference speaker and has worked with hundreds of trade and professional associations and universities. He has been a guest lecturer at Stanford University's Graduate School of Business and the University of Pennsylvania's Wharton School.

Don has also had extensive experience in the self-help publishing industry and sold one of his companies to Prentice Hall. His first book, *Up Your OWN Organization!*, was adopted by more than 150 universities. One of his companies published a 12-volume anthology of inspirational and self-help messages titled *Build a Better You—Starting Now!* that sold tens of thousands of copies. And he published *Chicken Soup for the Soul®* series creator Mark Victor Hansen's first book, *Future Diary*, 20 years ago.

Because of his extensive knowledge of the publishing industry, his experience as the author/editor/compiler/publisher of more than 40 books, his ability to work quickly and effectively with professional associations outside his own specialty areas, and his more than 65 years' experience as a model dental patient, the Chicken Soup organization asked Don to serve as co-author of *Chicken Soup for the Dental Soul*. Currently, Don's company, DMD House, and its distributors—several major dental supply houses—are the only sources through which *Chicken Soup for the Dental Soul* may be purchased.

Love Is the Best Medicine™ for Dental Patients and the Dental Team is the natural extension of Don's experience with *Chicken Soup for the Dental Soul*. This new book is available through major dental supply houses, Internet book retailers such as barnesandnoble.com and amazon.com and, of course, direct through DMD House.

To schedule Don for a presentation at your conference or meeting, please contact:

DMD House
29925 Rose Blossom Drive
Suite 300
Murrieta, CA 92563-4735

Phone: 909.677.6300
Fax: 909.698.0180
Email: dondible@dmdhouse.net
Website: www.dmdhouse.net

Richard H. Madow, DDS

One of dentistry's most prolific and beloved writers, Richard H. Madow, DDS, is co-founder of The Madow Group, a company whose mission is to help dentists, health professionals, and business owners enhance their practice or business, get more fulfillment from their work, and enjoy their lives as much as possible.

Founded with his brother, David M. Madow, DDS, in 1989, The Madow Group has grown from a two-man kitchen-table operation to an international publishing, educational, and marketing business with more than 30 employees and more than 20,000 clients in 12 countries. They are best known for *The Richards Report* dental newsletter, *The Richards Report* Cassette Tape Series, *The Richards Report* Super Fall Seminar—dentistry's largest privately held seminar, Promail Marketing, and many other uniquely designed products and services.

Rich is known throughout the dental community for his people skills and a sense of humor that lends itself to the entertainment provided at the annual Richards Report Seminar. It is the only meeting in dentistry where—besides finding the world's greatest dental, motivational, business, and lifestyle speakers—you will find dentists and their entire teams standing, singing, and dancing in the aisles to crazy dental parody songs, skits, and videos. The three-day event draws the finest, most enthusiastic dental offices from around the world and is often referred to as "T.B.S.E."—The Best Seminar Ever.

Rich lives in Owings Mills, Maryland, with his wife, Anne, and their two children, Michelle and Steven. He is an avid musician and musicologist, playing the piano, guitar, and various other instruments, and can often be seen on his front porch strumming a six-string and attempting to sing. His strange fascination with, and knowledge of, rock and roll trivia has yet to be explained.

For further information about The Madow Group, or to contact Rich, please try:

The Madow Group   Phone: 410.526.4780
230 Business Center Drive   Fax: 410.526.5186
Reisterstown, MD 21136   Email: rich@madow.com
Website: www.madow.com

Pamela Arbuckle Alston, DDS, FACD, graduated from the University of California at Berkeley and the University of California, San Francisco, School of Dentistry. Married to Rodrick Alston, she lives in the city where she was born—Oakland, California, and she works in Oakland, California, with her dental assistant, Janetta Barber. She counts as her children her nephews, nieces, stepdaughter, and patients at the Central Health Center. She thanks her mother, Ruby Arbuckle, eight sisters and brothers, and her friend, Ann Flinn, for listening to her many stories over the years about her patients and helping her to glean the lessons. And she gives God the glory for everything!

Kathleen E. Banas, RDH, has been a dental hygienist since 1981 and is part of the dental team of Neil Biederman, DDS. She also enjoys working at St. Isidore Church with youths from the sixth through the twelfth grades. Kathy's writing is both a hobby and a therapy; and her work has been published in *Marriage Encounter Magazine, Catholic Parent,* and *Woman's Day.* A Michigan resident, she shares life, love, and four wonderful teenage children—Maureen, Dan, Lindsay, and Gabriel—with Dan, her husband of 23 years. She is currently working on a book with her sister, Karen, about the trials and delights of raising teens. You may contact Kathy at Kat_E_blue7@yahoo.com.

Paul A. Bonstead, DDS, graduated from the University of Iowa in 1963 and then moved to France where he spent four years with the U.S. Army Dental Corps. He has provided volunteer dental services in many Third World and underdeveloped countries including Haiti, Honduras, and Mexico. He lectures frequently at dental meetings on practice management and has authored several articles for *Dental Economics* magazine. Married 38 years, Dr. Bonstead has three children and enjoys flower gardening and landscaping as a hobby. He practices general dentistry in St. Louis, Missouri, and can be reached by phone at 314.434.7887.

Elizabeth Ann Brandenburg, DA, resides in Rising Sun, Maryland, where her husband, Dr. Charles Lawrence Brandenburg, Jr., has practiced dentistry for 45 years. Elizabeth has studied at the Guilford Institute, Johns Hopkins University, and Lancaster Bible College. Lawrence is past president of the Maryland State Dental Association, and Elizabeth is past president of the Alliance of the Maryland State Dental Association. In partnership with her husband, Elizabeth has worked in affiliation with the Christian Medical and Dental Association, Flying Dentists, Wycliffe Bible Translators, JAARS, CBN, and Medical Missions International. Travel in service to the indigenous tribes of the world has taken Elizabeth to Mexico, Nicaragua, Guatemala, Haiti, Brazil, Equador, Chile, Kenya, Ethiopia, Zambia, Romania, Israel—and Madagascar.

Noel Brandon-Kelsch, RDH, a hygienist for ten years, has been married to the man of her dreams for 23 years. She has four wonderful children, Serena 22, Brice 20, Ma'rhya (Moe) 18, and DJ 17 (her foster son). She cradles people in her lap in the private practice of Dr. Philip Wolff in Marina, California. She received the ADHA "Bright Smiles, Bright Futures Award" and *USA* magazine's "National Make a Difference Day Award" in 2001 for all her volunteer efforts. If you would like to donate to, or help with, her volunteer sealant program and her efforts to help improve community oral health, Noel can be reached at Owellnoel@aol.com or at 831.455.9511.

Robin Brenner, RDH, graduated in 1981 from the Forsyth School for Dental Hygienists in Boston. In addition to practicing dental hygiene, she enjoys acting and wrote a one-woman show she has performed in New York and Los Angeles. She is most grateful for the wonderful people that have enhanced her life through her practice and that, in turn, she could brighten their smiles.

Diane Brucato-Thomas, RDH, EF, BS, founded the Hawai'i Institute for Wellness in Dentistry, has been a periodontal hygienist since 1979, served as anesthesia examiner for WREB, recorder for Hawaii BDE, clinical instructor for NAU, and vice president of ASDHA. HDHA awarded her "1999 Outstanding Member of the Year." Diane is currently vice president of WHDHA and first recipient of the Rosie Wall Community Spirit Grant from ADHA Oral Institute. She was previously published in *Chicken Soup for the Soul: A Fourth Course*. Married to a pharmacist, she has a son who is a unicycling fire juggler! Diane can be reached at PO Box 2065, Pahoa, HI 96778.

Mitchell J. Burgin, DDS, graduated from New York University and received his dental degree from the University of Maryland Dental School in 1949. After his orthodontic training at the University of Pennsylvania and two years in the U.S. Army Dental Corps, he practiced orthodontics in an area surrounded by the Berkshire Mountains of Massachusetts and the Green Mountains of Vermont. Now retired, he claims that serving young patients was what kept him young!

Julie Burton, RDH, has been a dental hygienist for 11 years and has served as a hygienist on several dental missions to Africa and Madagascar. Traveling is one of her passions, as are dabbling with writing and photography. She currently works for a general dentist in Coronado, California. Julie can be reached at Julietnan@aol.com.

Shari Caplan, RDH, graduated from the University of Pennsylvania School of Dental Hygiene in 1982 and worked for 15 years in her father's general practice, as well as for several pedodontists. Shari and husband, Jerry, have two great kids, Ashley, 13, and Blake, 9. Currently, Shari is co-owner of Security CPR Professionals with her sister, Amy. Their company provides CPR instruction, OSHA update courses and first aid training to the dental community, day-care personnel, and the lay public in their area. Shari resides in Owings Mills, Maryland, with her family. She can be reached at caplan86@aol.com.

Andrew Christopher, BS, DDS, MHA, FICD, is a retired associate professor from the Georgetown University School of Dentistry where he was the founding chairman of the Department of Community Dentistry. He has lectured widely on the history of dentistry and is past president of the American Academy of the History of Dentistry. Dr. Christopher is currently a Life Member of the District of Columbia Dental Society and the American Dental Association, and he is a Life Fellow of the International College of Dentists.

J. Walter Coffey, DDS, FAGD, FASDC, was born and grew up in Shawnee, Oklahoma. After completing undergraduate studies at Oklahoma University, he graduated in 1965 from the Baylor College of Dentistry. He went on to complete a one-year internship in the USAF followed by a two-year tour of duty at Perrin AFB. He has practiced general dentistry in Stillwater, Oklahoma, since 1968. He serves on the OAGD board of directors and is editor of the OAGD newsletter, *Impressions*. Dr. Coffey and his wife of 41 years, Diane, have four daughters and 13 grandchildren. You may contact him at jwcoffey2@aol.com.

Mary A. Cole, RDH, was born and raised in Rumford, Maine. She moved to Virginia in 1989 and graduated from Virginia Western College in 1995 with a degree in dental hygiene. Currently, she is employed by two general dental practices, one in Appomattox and the other in Lynchburg, Virginia.

S.G. Cooley is a poet, songwriter, and essayist. A native Virginian, the writer celebrates life in the Pacific Northwest with Ray, her husband of three decades, and their sons, John and Peter. She may be reached at sgcooley@integrity.com

Janice M. Dionis, RDH, was born and grew up in Worcester, Massachusetts. She began her dental career at the age of 16, working after school for an oral surgeon. She graduated from dental assisting school in 1978 and received her degree in dental hygiene from Quinsigamond Community College in 1991. In her 25 years in the dental field, she has worked as a receptionist, assistant, and hygienist in periodontal, pedodontal, and general practices. Currently, she works in a general and periodontal practice. She and her husband, Michael, have a son, Matthew, 19, a sophomore at Pennsylvania State University, and a daughter, Kaitlin, 17, a senior in high school.

Thomas G. Dwyer, DDS, MS, graduated from the Loma Linda University School of Dentistry in 1974. After three years in general dental practice, he returned to study in the graduate endodontic program. He earned a master of science degree in 1979 and has been in full-time private endodontic practice since then. In 1983, he completed the requirements for board certification and is a Diplomate of the American Board of Endodontics.

Bert F. Engstrom, DMD, graduated from Washington University School of Dental Medicine in 1985. He then completed a general practice residency at the University of Utah in 1986. He now practices general dentistry in Selma, California, with his twin brother. Dr. Engstrom is married and the father of six daughters.

Adrian Fenderson, DDS, has been practicing dentistry in northern California for 30 years. He has been a member of LMV for 20 years averaging over two missions a year. He is a decorated Vietnam veteran and has been a pilot since 1969. He can be reached at info@napadentist.com or through www.flyingdocs.org.

Sherrie L. Frame, RDH, has been a dental hygienist for 23 years and specialized in the treatment of periodontal disease for 15 years. She has enjoyed a varied career providing prevention programs for corporations, seminars for general dental offices, and public-health programs for schools and communities. She and her husband have three children and enjoy raising and training horses. Her hobbies include reading, cooking, running, and biking. The Frame family is in the process of selling their farm in Wisconsin and relocating to their second home in the Cody, Wyoming area.

Chris Freyermuth, DMD, has enjoyed 15 years in dentistry, graduating from the Tufts University School of Dental Medicine in 1986. He is available to patients throughout his local community via portable dental equipment in addition to maintaining a private practice in Plymouth, Massachusetts. Dr. Freyermuth's professional affiliations include AAA, AACD, IAO, AAFO, and AOS. He is personally unaffiliated. He can be reached via email at cfreyermuth@hotmail.com.

Danelle Fulawka, RDA, graduated in 1979 from the dental assisting program at Red River College in Winnipeg, Manitoba, Canada. After working several years in various private practices, she relocated to Calgary. In 1988, she accepted a position as Educational Technologist (Clinic Coordinator) with the Southern Alberta Institute of Technology, a dental assisting school, and has been employed there ever since. While at SAIT, she has continued her education, earning certificates in both management and marketing. In addition to her work at SAIT, Danelle currently serves as president of the

Canadian Dental Assistants Association, representing 19,000 dental assistants across Canada.

Jeffrey M. Galler, DDS, MAGD, lectures frequently at dental meetings, has authored articles in various dental journals, and holds patents in the field of restorative and cosmetic dentistry. In July 1999, he received the award of Master in the Academy of General Dentistry. Dr. Galler maintains a private practice in Brooklyn, New York.

Donald L. Gary, DDS, FAGD, is a 1973 graduate of the University of Tennessee College of Dentistry. He practices in Memphis (Germantown), Tennessee, is a Fellow in the Academy of General Dentistry, and was selected as Tennessee "Dentist of the Year" by that organization. Other memberships include the American Academy of Cosmetic Dentistry, Academy of Sports Dentistry, and the American Academy of Dental Practice Administration. He frequently lectures to dental organizations on topics including practice management and dental insurance. Dr. Gary may be contacted at 901.755.4132.

John R. Grasso, DDS, was born and raised in Binghamton, New York. He took his undergraduate and graduate degrees from the University of Southern California. At the age of 34, Dr. Grasso graduated from the Georgetown University School of Dentistry—Class of 1990. He then returned to Binghamton and, in addition to his private practice, created United Dental Services to serve the needy. United Dental Services was included in the U.S. Department of Health and Human Services 1996 edition of *Models That Work* a compendium of innovative primary healthcare programs for underserved and vulnerable populations. Dr. Grasso may be contacted by phone at 607.722.5929.

Jeffrey C. Gray, DDS, graduated from UCSF in 1986 and entered private practice with his wonderful Mary, a hygienist, in 1988. His loves include his two children, Jamie and Kyle, dentistry, and continuing to learn more about this thing called Life. In 1998, he created a program called "Smiles for Life" with the help of an incredible group of dental teams known as the Crown Council. Smiles for Life has raised and donated over $10 million to help children battling catastrophic illnesses. Last year the Crown Council teamed with superstar entertainer Garth Brooks and major league baseball for the benefit of even more children worldwide. Jeff can be reached at jgraydds@aol.com.

Kenneth Grubbs, DDS, received his BS from the University of Georgia at Athens in 1950 and his DDS from the Emory University School of Dentistry in 1956. He then opened a practice in Monroe, Georgia, situated one floor above a fish market. After 17 years, he moved to his present location—two blocks away—in a remodeled 160-year-old house. Dr. Grubbs flew his first airplane, a Piper J3 Cub, at the age of 15 and soloed at 16. He presently flies ultra-lights when he's not building and flying free-flight, contest model planes. He can be reached at kengdds@alltel.net.

Sheila Hall, DDS, graduated from the Loyola University School of Dentistry in 1987. She continued her specialty training in pediatric dentistry at Loyola University and Michigan's Mott Children's Health Center and Hurley Hospital. Dr. Hall is a Diplomate of the American Board of Pediatric Dentistry and has worked at the Infant Welfare Society of Chicago since completing her residency in 1989. She is married and resides in Lake Zurich, a suburb of Chicago. She can be reached at 1931 North Halsted Street, Chicago, IL 60614 or by phone at 312.751.2800.

Robert J. Harland, DMD, is a native Oregonian. Born in Dallas, Oregon, he grew up on his father's farm in Pickreall. He is a graduate of the College at the University of Oregon in Eugene and the University of Oregon School of Dentistry in Portland. He spent three years in the U.S. Navy as a dental officer on the aircraft carrier Lexington. He then opened a private general practice in Eugene that he operated for 28 years. Dr. Harland was in the mission field for six years in Africa and now works for an HMO in Eugene.

D. Michael Hart, DDS, FAGD, MAGD, received his DDS from Columbia University in 1980. He continued his education with a one-year general practice residency and numerous continuing education courses. Dr. Hart has been awarded both the Fellowship and the Mastership in the AGD. He founded a group dental practice that currently has four dentists including an orthodontist. Dr. Hart is a member of the ADA and serves on the staff of the JFK Medical Center. Married, with two children, his hobbies include fly-fishing, golf, and skiing. Dr. Hart may be contacted at Gentle Dental Care, LLC, 2060 Oak Tree Road, Edison, NJ 08820 or by phone at 732.549.5660.

Karen L. Hart-Sabol, RDH, is a 1990 dental hygiene graduate of the State University of New York in Farmingdale, Long Island. She attended Michael Schuster's Center for Professional Development in Scottsdale, Arizona, and has been a full-time practicing hygienist for 11 years in northern New Jersey. She presently works in the office of Kevin Dougherty, DMD, who utilizes the Pankey Institute philosophy. She has been married three wonderful years to her husband, Jeff, and they are the proud parents of a son, Logan Davis, born on April 3, 2001. The Sabols share their home in New Vernon, New Jersey, with a dog named Tanner.

Leanne Haynes, RDH, BS, lives in a small town in southern Tennessee with her husband, Mike, and their four-legged companion, Butler. Since graduation from the University of Tennessee in 1978, she has practiced dental hygiene in the same office with a team she regards as her second family. Her favorite aspect of hygiene has been establishing and maintaining relationships with long-standing patients. She also operates a small decorative sewing business and, with Mike, enjoys scouting for—and collecting—old toys.

Mandy Hayre-Dhasi, RDH, BDSc, PID, is married to a wonderful man, Paul, and has two beautiful children named Travis and Jaslyn. She lives in Nanaimo, British Columbia, on Vancouver Island in Canada. She is an educator at Malaspina University-College and is also a masters of education student at the University of Victoria. She practices as a clinical dental hygienist in general and periodontal specialty offices. Mandy would like to thank her parents, Avtar and Manjit Hayre in Quesnel, British Columbia, and her in-laws, Tarsem and Bahkshish Dhasi in Nanaimo, British Columbia, for their exceptional support during her life! She may be contacted at dhasim@mala.bc.ca.

Charles S. Horn, III, DDS, was born and raised in Rehobeth Beach, Delaware, graduated from the University of Delaware, and still considers himself a small-town boy. He received his DDS in 1961 from the Temple University School of Dentistry and graduated in the top ten percent of his class. After a stretch in the U.S. Army, he set up practice in Wilmington, Delaware. He was never president of his state dental association nor held any other such high position. In the story, "Bomb Squad," you will understand why Dr. Horn loves dentistry and enjoys Life—especially fly-fishing, cooking, and a good joke. His fax number is 302.478.3437.

Allyson K. Hurley, DDS, MAGD, AACD, has a restorative-cosmetic dentistry practice in Chatham, New Jersey. Dr. Hurley received her master's degree in the AGD in 1993, and became accredited in the AACD in 2001. She has the distinction of being one of only two women in the world to have attained this honor. She enjoys time spent with her family, walking on the beach, and nature photography. Her passion for photography has spilled over into teaching oral and portrait photography to her colleagues. Dr. Hurley feels strongly that helping others is its own reward and supports numerous charities.

Mohamed Hussein, DDS, graduated from the University of Western Ontario with a major in genetics and then attended the University of Toronto Faculty of Dentistry. Since receiving his degree in 1989, Dr. Hussein worked in private practice and with children at the Ministry of Health. In 1995, Dr. Hussein, his wife, and two children moved to Guelph, and he took over his present practice. Dr. Hussein also teaches at the University of Western Ontario and dedicates his story, "Marital Status," to the giants on whose shoulders he has been able to reach further heights—his parents. You are invited to visit his Website at www.guelphdentistry.com.

Cathy Jameson, PhD, is president of Jameson Management, Inc., an international dental lecture and consulting firm. An accomplished speaker, writer, and workshop leader, Cathy holds a PhD in psychology, where she focused her work on effective, stress-controlled management. Her 25 years of "hands-on" experience in her husband's dental practice makes her strategies workable and effective. Cathy has been a featured speaker for the major dental meetings throughout the world and is also an adjunct faculty member of the Oklahoma University School of Dentistry. Cathy divides her time between her travels around the world and her horse ranch in southern Oklahoma.

Helen Jasnosz, DDS, graduated from the Case Western Reserve University School of Dentistry. She practices dentistry in New York State where she lives with her teenage children, Tess and Will. Her story reverses the theme of this book. "Sam Eagle" is not the story of a doctor with a heart. It is, instead, the story of a patient with a heart. Her life has been enriched, and her horizons expanded, by the thoughtful care her patients have given her.

Gregory R. Johnson, DDS, is a graduate of Virginia Tech and received his dental degree in 1989 at the Medical College of Virginia. Currently, he practices general dentistry in Charleston, South Carolina, where he resides with his wife, Vicki, and two beautiful daughters, Caroline and Hannah. Dr. Johnson enjoys boating, fishing, golf, and following Hokie football.

Harry T. Keyes, DDS, graduated from the University of Washington School of Dentistry in 1959 and immediately passed the board exams for Washington, Oregon, and Nevada. After spending a year in each of two group practices, he opened his own general dentistry practice in Pasco, Washington, in 1961. Today, he and his two associates serve more than 10,000 patients. When not practicing dentistry, Dr. Keyes may often be found at the eyepiece of his Meade 12" LX200 Schmidt-Cassegrain telescope studying the night sky. You may contact his office at 888.DR.KEYES.

Christy Ellis King, RDH, RDA, has a degree in zoology from the University of Arkansas and a degree in dental hygiene from the University of Arkansas for Medical Sciences. She has the opportunity of working for her husband, Mitchell D. King, DDS. Their practice, King Family Dental Care, is located in Christy's hometown of Conway, Arkansas. Currently, Christy stays at home with their son, Haydon. She handles the practice's insurance, billing, and collections from home. The story "Taking a Bite Out of Crime" is based on the life of the late father of Mitch's University of Tennessee Dental School roommate, Wade W. Robertson.

April Klepper, RDH, has been a hygienist for 12 years. She works part-time and enjoys cooking, antique shopping, and church activities. She, her husband, Monty, and their five-year-old daughter, Hope, live in Oklahoma City, Oklahoma.

Debby Kurtz-Weidinger, RDH, MEd, has been a faculty member at Phoenix College's Dental Hygiene Program since 1984, and she is also a public-health dental hygienist with the Arizona State Health Department, Office of Oral Health. Debby has been actively involved in the design and development of Internet-based instruction for dental professionals since obtaining her master's degree in instructional technology. She considers her greatest accomplishment, however, to be the successful raising of her two teenage sons, Andrew and Kevin, with the help of Joe, her husband of 25 years.

Deborah D. Landis, RDH, a U.S. Navy veteran, majored in biology at Cal State and is also a graduate of the University of Texas. She holds licenses to practice in Texas, Florida, and California. Recently relocating to Olathe Kansas, Deborah is pursuing her licensure there. Having been raised in Illinois, she is glad to be back in the Midwest, after all, "There is no place like home!" She can be reached at Landisdd@aol.com.

Stanley J. Larsen, DDS, FAGD, passed away in January 2001 at the age of 48 after succumbing to renal cancer. Following his graduation from the University of Iowa College of Dentistry in 1977, Dr. Larsen established a successful general practice in Watertown, Wisconsin. A dentist highly respected by his patients and his professional colleagues, he was also very active in his community in the Chamber of Commerce, the Jaycees, and the Rotary Club and his church, the United Methodist Church, where he served on several committees. He served as president of the Watertown United Way and, an Eagle Scout, he was also a scout-master. Dr. Larsen was an avid sports and hobby enthusiast who enjoyed tennis, canoeing, hiking, water and snow skiing, camping, photography, woodworking, and ham radio. A loving husband and father, Dr. Larsen is survived by his wife, Vicki, and their four children, Jennifer, Jason, Danielle, and Brianna.

Robert E. Lavine, DDS, graduated from the University of Michigan School of Dentistry in 1964. Following a two-year tour of duty in the U.S. Air Force, he opened his dental practice in Warren, Michigan. Three weeks later, he met Bylaina who would become his wife and office manager for 34 years and counting. The Lavines have a son, Gary, who is a senior scientist with Beyond Genomics in Boston, and a daughter, Sherri, who is a merchandise planner with the KMart Corporation. Dr. Lavine is a member of the Michigan Dental Association Forensic Dental Identification Team.

Marla Leibfried, CDA, has been in the dental field since 1976. In addition to her work in a private practice, she teaches dental assisting at a local technical college. Marla lives in southwest Wisconsin with her husband, Doug, who farms, and their two children, Jenny and Nick. Marla's family has always been very supportive of her motivation for, and admiration of, the "drill and fill" profession.

Judee Limardi, RDH, grew up in Westchester, Illinois. She attended Marquette University, receiving a certificate in dental hygiene and a BS in 1977. She has practiced as a clinical dental hygienist for 25 years, with the last 15 at Hawthorn Dental Associates in Vernon Hills. She particularly enjoys visiting schools to talk to children about their teeth. Her long career in private practice has given Judee the opportunity to meet many fascinating people and prompted her to write stories about her experiences in the dental office. She has two children, D.J. and Katie. Judee can be reached at Toothee126@aol.com.

Ann Madigan, DMD, MSc, specialist in pediatric dentistry, is a past president of the White Plains (New York) Dental Forum, and founding dentist of Westchester Pediatric Dentistry PC. She is a frequent lecturer on topics related to providing dental care for children. Dr. Madigan is a contributing editor to a pediatric medical journal and the mother of two grown-as-they'll-get boys. Her Website is www.kids-dentist.com.

Ira Marder, DDS, FAGD, graduated from the University of Toronto Faculty of Dentistry in 1987 as a Doctor of Dental Surgery and, in 2000, received his Fellowship from the Academy of General Dentistry. Ira has been a clinical instructor at the University of Toronto and a president of the Alpha Omega Dental Society. As well, he has been very involved in numerous dental, charitable, social, and cultural organizations. Currently, he maintains two practices in Toronto, Canada, where he lives with his family. Ira dedicates his story "Wasted Effort" to the Ebidia-Wiseman families.

John McCormack, DDS, graduated in dentistry from Guys Hospital in London and later obtained his DDS from the University of Toronto in Canada. He is a past president of the British Society for Restorative Dentistry and of the American Dental Society of London. He has taught and lectured on restorative dentistry and operates a private practice in Harley Street, London. In addition to making regular fly-fishing trips from Russia to Patagonia, he maintains a resource Website for dental graphics at www.dentagraphics.co.uk.

Amy M. McLamb is a graduate of Peace College in Raleigh, North Carolina, and earned a BA in Communication from North Carolina State University. For the past ten years, she has been a practice administrator for Dr. Mark

Odom, an endodontist, in Cary, North Carolina, where she lives with her wonderful husband, Mike, and their Labrador retriever, Shasta. She is a member of PAHCOM (Professional Association of Health Care Office Managers), enjoys walking, biking, and hiking, and is active in her community. Amy takes this opportunity to dedicate her story, "Credit Report," to her parents, Anne and Vance Miller, for "raising her right" with their love and support.

Sharon Melanson, RDH, graduated from the University of Alberta in 1979 and has spent her career in public health. She has participated in several research projects including work with several Native Bands, studies on the high incidence of early childhood caries (ECC) among First Nations groups, and the health effects of using smokeless tobacco. Sharon lives on a farm in Armstrong, British Columbia, with her husband and two sons and works as a community dental hygienist for the Okanagan Similkameen Health Region. She would like to have some hobbies, but with her job, her two active boys, and helping run the farm, she hasn't found the time!

Cathy Milejczak, CDA, RDH, BHS, hails from Columbia, South Carolina. She and her husband, Vic, are active members of the Trinity Lutheran Church. Together they share three children. She works for Midlands Technical College as the compliance specialist and lab manager for the Health Sciences Department and does part-time clinical hygiene with Dr. Bill Flemming. Cathy enjoys reading, sewing, and traveling. She has participated with four dental mission teams serving in Kenya, Tanzania, and Romania. She feels blessed to have a wonderful family, friends, and coworkers who encourage her with all her adventures. Cathy can be reached at czaks@aol.com.

Linda Miles, CSP, CMC, has become an icon in the dental management arena during the past 22 years. Her prestigious consulting firm, Dental Dynamics, Inc., was listed by *Inc.* magazine as one of the fastest-growing privately held companies in America in 1987. She has lectured in all 50 states, at every major meeting, and on four continents. Her insight into the humanistic side of managing people and growing successful businesses has made her the mentor to more than 100 other speakers and consultants.

Betty Moss, CDA, was born in 1931 in Washington State near the Canadian border. She graduated from high school in Santa Maria, California, and then attended the Dental Nurses Training School in San Francisco from which she graduated in 1951. Married soon after, she and her husband moved to Chapel Hill, North Carolina, where she worked with handicapped children as a dental assistant at the University of North Carolina School of Dentistry for ten years. She then moved to the UNC

Hospital Dental Clinic and served adult hemophilia patients for ten years. Until her recent retirement at age 70, Betty worked in the office of Charles Arnett, DDS, in North Myrtle Beach.

Sandra C. Nelson, RDH, BS, LAP, graduated from the Oregon Health Sciences University with a dental hygiene certificate in 1967. She completed her degree program in 1991 at the Southern Oregon State College. After 34 years of private practice, she has started her own limited-access business, Smiles All Around, providing dental hygiene services to those living in assisted residential care facilities. She can be reached at cowgirlrising@msn.com.

Rudi Neumarker, DDS, received his BS in zoology from Brigham Young University and graduated from the University of California, San Francisco School of Dentistry in 1970. He began his career in a group practice owned by his father-in-law where he worked for four years before buying an established general dentistry practice in Palo Alto, California. He and his wife, Leslie, live in Menlo Park and have five children, Nicole, Melissa, Todd, Joshua, and Margan, and one grandchild, Brynlee. When he is not practicing dentistry, Dr. Neumarker enjoys restoring old homes. You may contact his Palo Alto office at 650.329.8160.

Steven Novick, DDS, works in the dental practice he always dreamed of owning in the wonderful town of Franklin Square, New York. He is a board member of the Nassau County Dental Society and is a firm believer in organized dentistry. His wife, Adrienne, and children, Peri, Max, and Teagan, have been very supportive of his dental pursuits, his writing, and his acting. Dr. Novick has appeared in the television series *Star Trek: Voyager* and *Star Trek: Deep Space Nine*. He has the most dedicated dental staff in the universe and counts himself lucky to work with such fine individuals. "One Winter" is dedicated to all his past and present patients who have made coming to work every day a challenge and a pleasure!

Sue O'Brien, RDH, graduated from the University of Minnesota as a dental hygienist in 1965. For the last 25 years, she has worked in a Minneapolis dental practice as an administrator in addition to her clinical hygiene duties. She loves every aspect of the dental practice but particularly values the relationships developed with patients and her fellow team members. Sue was a charter Editorial Board Member of *RDH* magazine, wrote a newsletter for the practice for 20 years, and designed and maintains a Website for the office. Sue's other great love is her family—husband Tom, four children and their spouses, and five grandchildren.

Mary M. O'Connor, DDS, is a graduate of the University of San Diego and the Loyola University School of Dentistry in Chicago, Illinois. She completed her specialty training in pediatric dentistry at Loyola with part of her training completed in a residency in Flint, Michigan. She maintains a private pediatric dental practice in San Diego, California, and devotes a large percentage of her practice to adults and children with special needs. Dr. O'Connor and her wonderful husband, John, have three children, twins Matthew and Patrick and their younger sister, Emily.

Tom Orent, DMD, is a management consultant and practicing dentist in Framingham, Massachusetts, and a past president of the New England Chapter of the American Academy of Cosmetic Dentistry. Dr. Orent has served on the faculty of Boston University's Goldman School of Dental Medicine and has been featured as a guest lecturer at dental schools across the nation. He has lectured to dentists in four countries and 46 of the 50 United States, and his books, tapes, and newsletters are sold in 20 countries. Chairperson of the Public Relations Committee for the AACD, he was accredited by that organization in 1990 and has served as editor of the *AACD Journal*. The author of four books and numerous articles on dentistry, Dr. Orent is considered to be one of the pioneers of "Instant Orthodontics."

Clyde T. Padgett, Jr., DDS, or "Shot," as he is known to his family and friends, has been practicing general dentistry in his hometown of Florence, South Carolina, for more than 38 years. He received his undergraduate degree from Wofford College in Spartanburg, South Carolina, and completed his dental training at the University of Virginia Dental College in 1963. He and his wife, Betsy, have three children and four grandchildren.

Richard L. Parker, DDS, MS, is a 1968 graduate of the Loma Linda University School of Dentistry. He received his master's degree in oral biology from the Medical College of Georgia in 1975. He was dental director of the Guam Seventh-Day Adventist Dental Clinic from 1968 to 1973. From 1973 to 1994 he was in dental education where he was the Assistant Professor of Oral Medicine at The Medical College of Georgia and Associate Professor of Oral Diagnosis at Loma Linda University School of Dentistry. Currently, Dr. Parker's family dental practice is in Calimesa, California.

Mary S. Pelletier, RDH, BS, resides in Port St. Lucie, Florida, with her husband, Jerry, and their two daughters, Michelle and Jeneé. Mary has been a registered dental hygienist for 20 years. She is an adjunct faculty member at Indian River Community College Dental Hygiene Program in Ft. Pierce, Florida, and works in private practice with Radamee Orlandi, DDS, in Jensen Beach, Florida. Mary enjoys sharing her dental hygiene experience with the students and keeping her skills fine-tuned in the general dental practice.

Jackie S. Perry, RDH, BSDH, worked as a dental assistant and dental hygienist in general dentistry practices for almost 30 years. Ms. Perry is now in the process of completing her master's degree in dental hygiene education while working as a graduate teacher's assistant in Old Dominion University's Dental Hygiene Program. She resides in Virginia with her husband and their 17-year-old son.

Richard L. Plasch, DDS, FAGD, was born and raised in Southern California. He is a graduate of the University of California, San Francisco School of Dentistry. After serving two years in the U.S. Air Force as a dentist, he opened his practice in Hayward, California. Dr. Plasch's efforts are concentrated in the area of restorative, preventive, and cosmetic dentistry. He is active in various dental organizations and is a past president of his local Rotary Club. Away from his practice and professional responsibilities, Dr. Plasch enjoys photography, snow skiing, and family activities.

Mary Jo Pletz, RDH, received a specialized diploma in dental assisting in 1993 at the age of 18 and began her dental career one week later in the office of Dr. Richard DiEdwardo with a focus on implantology. For the next six years, she attended school at night and received her dental hygiene degree from Northampton Community College in 1999. Mary Jo has been married to her wonderful husband, John, for five years, and they have a ten-month-old son, Douglas. Her hobbies include photography, crafts, and gardening.

Steven L. Rasner, DMD, MAGD, earned his dental degree from the University of Pennsylvania School of Dental Medicine in 1980 and received the award of Master in the Academy of General Dentistry in 1997. He shares the rewards of his practice with his wife, June, and their three children. The author of a lecture series designed to empower dental professionals, Dr. Rasner speaks to more than 5,000 dental team members every year. His lecture series, "Realizing the Dream," reveals the protocols and philosophies that fire the success of his Bridgeton, New Jersey, practice. For more information and a schedule of presentations, please email DrRasner@aol.com.

Bess Reeverts, CDA, RDA, has enjoyed an 18-year career in dentistry. A graduate of Lansing Community College, she is past president of the Central District Dental Assistants Association and has served on the Michigan Dental Assistants Association as nominating committee chair, corresponding secretary, and recording secretary. She is a recipient of the Ruth M. Edwards Award and has served on the Lansing Community College Dental Board for three terms. For the past five years, she has worked in the office of Tim Chapel, DDS, in Jackson, Michigan. Bess and her husband, Dave, have two daughters and two grandchildren. Bess enjoys gardening as a hobby.

Robert Reyto, DDS, FAACD, graduated from Tufts College in 1959 and earned his dental degree from the Case Western Reserve University School of Dentistry in 1963. He is a Fellow of the American Academy of Cosmetic Dentistry and the Academy of General Dentistry and holds a Certificate in Laser Tooth Whitening. You may reach Dr. Reyto's Beverly Hills office at 310.275.1137.

Naomi Rhode, RDH, CSP, CPAE Speaker Hall of Fame, is an Alumnus of the Year, University of Minnesota Dental School; a past president of the Arizona Dental Hygienists Association; a past president of the National Speakers Association; and a co-founder of SmartPractice. For over 27 years she has graced healthcare and business platforms with her presentations on leadership, communication, teamwork, balance, and empowerment. She is a wife, mother, and grandmother of 12. Naomi is currently serving on many national boards of directors and is the author of two books, *More Beautiful Than Diamonds: The Gift of Friendship* and *The Gift of Family: A Legacy of Love*. She is the co-author of *Meditations for Road Warriors*, contributing author to 20 other books, and producer of CD/cassette programs on marriage and on practice team/patient communication. You may contact Naomi at SmartPractice, 3400 E. McDowell Road, Phoenix, AZ 85006, 800.522.0595, x 214, nrhode@smarthealth.com, or www.smartpractice.com.

Robert E. Riddle, DDS, is a graduate of Wittenberg University and received his dental degree in 1969 from Indiana University. He immediately returned to his hometown of Goshen, Indiana, to continue his father's dental practice. His wife, Carolynn, whom he met in dental school, volunteered to "help out" until a new office manager could be hired. Thirteen years later, she still runs the office and has been told she needs to give at least five years' notice if she ever wants to quit! The Riddles have one son, Jeff, who is an engineer and a captain in the U.S. Air Force, and a yellow Labrador retriever, Shelby. Dr. Riddle enjoys writing, photography, and traveling. Dr. Riddle's office may be reached by calling 219.875.6169.

Nancy Roe-Pimm, RDH, works with a wonderful dentist, Dr. Jim Nicholls, and his awesome staff—Sandie, Karen, Cindy, Jen, Jodi, and Jacquie. Nancy and Ed, her husband of 24 years, have three beautiful daughters, Ali, Lindsay, and Carli. She graduated from New York's Orange County Community College and has worked as a dental hygienist for 21 years. Nancy is also a freelance writer and an animal lover with three dogs, three cats, and four horses. She offers special thanks to Kathy Kane for encouraging her to submit the stories appearing in this book. You may reach Nancy at npimm@aol.com.

Rhonda R. Savage, DDS, graduated with honors from the University of Washington School of Dentistry in 1989. After three years as a dental officer in the U.S. Navy, she purchased a private practice in Tacoma, Washington. She is a member of the Pierre Fauchard Academy and the International College of Dentists. Rhonda is past president of Pierce County Dental Society and is on the board of directors of the Washington State Dental Association. She is on the board of directors of the Point Defiance Zoo and volunteers as the "zoo dentist." She can be reached at savage@harbornet.com.

Joanne Iannone Sheehan, RDH, grew up in East Hampton, New York, and graduated from SUNY at Farmingdale in 1974. She has practiced dental hygiene in five states and Germany due to her husband's military career. Her two children are currently attending high school and college. A frequent contributor to *RDH* magazine since 1997, Joanne is most known for her humorous renditions of "Life in the Dental Lane." (Her parents are responsible for her unusual sense of humor.) She can be reached at 111 Windingham Drive, Huntsville, AL 35806.

Sherwin Shinn, DDS, graduated from the University of Washington Dental School in 1974 and currently maintains a private practice in Issaquah, Washington. He and his wife, Jerri, an RN, have two wonderful sons, Josef and Michael, and have co-founded the nonprofit "International Smile Power Foundation," which delivers health care, supplies, and disease prevention education to developing countries where there is little or no access to care. Dr. Shinn is an inspirational speaker and the entertaining author of *Confessions of a Modern Dentist* from which his excerpts in this book are taken. For more information about his dental outreach adventures, please check www.smilepower.org.

Robert C. Smithwick, DDS, FACD, graduated from the University of Illinois College of Dentistry and served as a U.S. Navy dental officer aboard ship in the Pacific during WWII. He later served as a dental officer to the Stewart Indian Agency and School in Nevada. Dr. Smithwick was on the clinical staff of what is now the UOP Dental School, served on the board of the California Dental Association, was a delegate to the 1956 White House Conference on Health, a member of the ADA, CDA, and AAPD, and a Fellow in the American College of Dentists. On retirement, he was awarded the 1987 Meritorious Service Award from the ACD. He served as an Assistant Director, Public Health, for the State of California from 1972 to 73. For the last 35 years of his career, he was a pediatric dentist.

Becky Sroda, RDH, MS, received her BS from the University of Detroit in 1974 and her MS from the University of Michigan in 1980. She has been in dental hygiene education for 21 years and is currently an instructor of dental hygiene at Asheville-Buncombe Technical Community College in Asheville, North Carolina, where she teaches oral health care (surprise), nutrition, and dental ethics. She enjoys writing short stories and sending them as letters to friends and family. In her spare time, she is helping her father write a book about his experience as a POW during WWII.

Ian W. Tester, DDS, practices dentistry in the Glendale Dental Centre, St. Catharines, Ontario, Canada. He is blessed with three wonderful children, Christopher, Lauren, and Jillian. Together, they enjoy many outdoor sports including hiking, cycling, and canoeing. Professionally, Ian is devoted to continuing education, studying, and lecturing on comprehensive dentistry.

Eric B. Wall, DDS, has practiced oral and maxillofacial surgery in the Stockton area since 1981. His career in private practice has been enhanced by his commitment to continuing education, his active involvement in local and national dental organizations, and his dedication to the community. After earning his dental degree from the University of California, San Francisco, School of Dentistry, he went on to receive his specialty degree in oral and maxillofacial surgery from the Los Angeles County/University of Southern California Medical Center. Dr. Wall enjoys spending time with his wife and his two children, Brandon and Lindsey. His hobbies include golf, snow skiing, and sailing.

Robert F. Weed, DDS, received his BS from Brigham Young University in 1975 and his DDS in 1979 from the Temple University School of Dentistry. He maintains a busy practice with his partner, Dr. David J. Probst, in Fallon, Nevada. Dr. Weed and his wife, Rebecca, are the parents of six children. "Becky and I love our role as parents. We recognize that the most significant work we do is within the circle of our family," says Dr. Weed. One son is following in his father's footsteps at the University of the Pacific School of Dentistry, while another son pursues a related degree at the University of Nevada School of Medicine.

Jane Weiner, RDH, graduated from the Forsyth School for Dental Hygienists in Boston in 1964. A practicing dental hygienist, she is an adjunct faculty member in the Periodontal Pre-doctoral Department of Nova SE College of Dental Medicine in Fort Lauderdale, Florida; owner of Jane Weiner, RDH, Board Reviews, Inc.; and a frequent contributor to *RDH* magazine. Jane resides in Tamarac, Florida, with her husband of 30 years. They have two wonderful children, one an occupational therapist and the other a music and band promoter. Jane can be reached at rdhjw@aol.com.

Lisa M. Wendell, DMD, was born and raised in Farmington, Connecticut, before moving to Boston, Massachusetts, to attend the Tufts University

School of Dental Medicine. After graduating in 1988, she furthered her education at Tufts in the Department of Endodontics. Lisa has been a member of the faculty at Tufts Dental School and has conducted continuing education seminars on the subject of endodontics. She is a partner in a multi-office endodontic practice west of Boston. She presently resides in Southborough, Massachusetts, with her husband, Ken Fishman, and three wonderful daughters, Carolyn, Andrea, and Dana.

Daniel E. White, DDS, graduated from the Indiana University School of Dentistry in 1979 and then entered a group general dentistry practice. In 1995, he and a partner opened a general dentistry practice, also in South Bend. Dr. White's story, "Once Again, Thank You," refers to his wife, Nancy, whose cancer continues in remission. His partner, Dr. Tim Kulik, who now has only one arm, recently placed a crown on one of Dr. White's teeth. Dr. White would like to take this opportunity to thank his extended family, his children, Andrew and Alison, and his loving and caring 15-member staff for their unstinting support through these difficult times.

Cheryl Lee Willett, DDS, MS, is a graduate of the University of Miami, Florida. She received her Doctor of Dental Surgery degree from Northwestern University in 1997. She then completed her specialty certificate in pediatric dentistry from the University of Maryland in 1999. She earned her MS in oral biology in 2001, also from the University of Maryland. She and her husband, Dr. Raymond Ramos, a fellow pediatric dentist, reside in northern California.

A.T. Williams, DDS, grew up in Miami, Florida, and is a graduate of the Baylor College of Dentistry in Dallas, Texas. He practiced in Coral Gables, Florida, a few blocks away from the office of Dr. L.D. Pankey, and was an early student of this great man before there was a Pankey Institute. Dr. Williams's interests and philosophy are products of Dr. Pankey's early teachings about "long centric," anterior guidance—the PMS technique. He enjoys a good game of golf, hot air ballooning, white water rafting, snorkeling, and tarpon fishing. After 37 years, quality dentistry—coupled with quality patient care—continues to be a major interest to him.

Linda Williams, RDH, resides in Latham, New York, and is employed by First Advantage Dental group practice at the office of Dr. Robert Brand in Delmar. Prior to working for Dr. Brand, she was employed for 20 years in the HMO environment. She and her husband, Doug, have raised six children and are now discovering the joy of being grandparents. Linda is proud of the role her career has played in dental and medical preventive care.

Ethel Wolff, RDH, born in New Jersey, has resided for 28 years in Ohio. A graduate of the University of Pennsylvania School of Dental Hygiene, she currently works part-time in a private practice. She also works on a dental sealant team that serves Akron's inner-city schools. She has been a volunteer on many school and religious committees and served as president of the support group of the Northern Ohio Chapter of the American Liver Foundation. Ethel lives with her husband, Marc, and their two daughters, Beth and Amy. She enjoys spending time with her family, cooking, traveling, and seeing New York's Broadway shows.

David Zamboni, RDH, BS, was born and raised in Lakewood, Colorado; however, he was told that he was conceived elsewhere! A former part-time hygiene instructor and a current practicing hygienist, David enjoys the endless personal rewards he receives through meeting and helping people on a daily basis. Outside of dental hygiene, he mentors troubled youths in the community. He is currently adjusting to life as a newlywed with the love of his life.